On Balance

On Balance

ADAM PHILLIPS

HAMISH HAMILTON
an imprint of
PENGUIN BOOKS

HAMISH HAMILTON

Published by the Penguin Group
Penguin Books Ltd, 80 Strand, London WC2R ORL, England
Penguin Group (USA) Inc., 375 Hudson Street, New York, New York 10014, USA
Penguin Group (Canada), 90 Eglinton Avenue East, Suite 700, Toronto, Ontario, Canada M4P 2Y3
(a division of Pearson Penguin Canada Inc.)
Penguin Ireland, 25 St Stephen's Green, Dublin 2, Ireland (a division of Penguin Books Ltd)
Penguin Group (Australia), 250 Camberwell Road, Camberwell, Victoria 3124, Australia
(a division of Pearson Australia Group Pty Ltd)
Penguin Books India Pvt Ltd, 11 Community Centre, Panchsheel Park, New Delhi – 110 017, India
Penguin Group (NZ), 67 Apollo Drive, Rosedale, North Shore 0632, New Zealand
(a division of Pearson New Zealand Ltd)
Penguin Books (South Africa) (Pty) Ltd, 24 Sturdee Avenue, Rosebank, Johannesburg 2196, South Africa

Penguin Books Ltd, Registered Offices: 80 Strand, London WC2R ORL, England

www.penguin.com

First published 2010

1

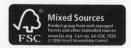

For Michel Gribinski and Michael Neve

... what counts as an accurate report
of experience is a matter of what a
community will let you get away with.

Richard Rorty, 'Cultural Politics and the
Question of the Existence of God'

Underneath the disability my inability was intact.

Adam Mars-Jones, *Pilcrow*

People unused to upholstered
furniture do not have a desire for it.

Keith Thomas, *The Ends of Life*

Contents

Preface

'There seems to be something singularly captivating in the word balance,' John Stuart Mill said in a talk to The Mutual Improvement Society in 1834, 'as if, because anything is called a balance, it must, for that reason, be necessarily good.' When we want a balanced economy, or a balance of power, or want people to make balanced judgements; when we describe disturbing people as unbalanced, or assume, as we are likely to do these days, that anyone who is troubled by anything is suffering from a chemical imbalance, we are promoting the image that Mill wants us to be wary of. That it is an image – a picture of something, of somebody creating a kind of order – and that we are beguiled by it is worth noting. Justice with her scales is infinitely reassuring; the man walking on wire between the Twin Towers is both horrifying and fascinating; and children, so soon after learning to walk, loving to go round and round in circles until they fall over is puzzling (the advantage of lying on the floor, Kafka remarked in his diary, is that there is nowhere else to fall). Balance, like all our fundamental things, is something we can find, keep, lose and use; it is something we often want. Because it is 'singularly captivating', Mill suggests, we think it must 'be necessarily good'. There is indeed nothing like it; but Mill thinks we should be suspicious of anything that might confine us by lulling us into a state of inattention.

We wouldn't put it quite like that now, but the people we fall in love with we find singularly captivating, as are any of the people (or ideas) that inspire us, for better or for worse. What is strange about Mill's simple observation is that it is the singularly captivating that tends to make us lose our balance. Mill intimates with his peculiar logic that the idea of balance can unbalance us. And yet in one traditional version of the moral life, as Mill knows, it is balance that is sought. Indeed, it was part of Mill's liberalism to believe that we should be able to 'enter into the mind and circumstance' of those with opposing views to our own. When the dramatist Mark Ravenhill writes that 'Art that isn't driven by this basic impulse to create an unbalanced view of the world is probably bad or weak,' we are not shocked by this, partly because after Romanticism we take it for granted that this is the province of art; elsewhere it is balance that is required. Art, ideally, is where the unbalanced views should be kept, as far away from religion and politics as possible. If we want art to be an isolation ward it is because we know just how contagious these so-called unbalanced views of the world can be (fascism, racism and sexism in modern liberal societies

are unbalanced views, but liberal democratic values
are not). It is of some significance that when we talk
about many of the things that matter most to us – as
the essays in this book on excess, on fundamentalism
and on schooling suggest – we soon lose our so-called
balanced views. So we should not, perhaps, underestimate our wish to lose our balance, even though
it's often easier to get up than to fall over. Indeed, the
sign that something does matter to us is that we lose
our steadiness.

The first psychoanalysts, who wanted to think of
themselves as scientists, considered psychoanalysis as
a kind of laboratory for the study of unbalanced views;
it wasn't long before they began to believe that everyone, including themselves, hadn't merely lost their
balance, they had never had it. And that everyone, by
nature, as it were, was in disarray, was riven with conflict. (They also tended to believe that psychoanalysis
was unequivocally a good thing when, on balance, it
is something about which we should always be
divided.) Like Mill, they began to realize that balance
– or more specifically the idea of the balanced mind
– was no longer a useful picture for modern people.
They asked us to ask why anyone would want to be a
well-balanced person: what were the conditions –
familial, political, economic – that might produce
this as an ideal? So the essays in this book are about
the balancing acts that modern societies involve us
in. Secular, liberal societies encourage their citizens

to believe that they might have some choice about what they find singularly captivating, and that they are capable of making balanced judgements. One of the things that psychoanalysis does is add something new to the long cultural conversation about what the phrase 'singularly captivating' might mean, and what judgement might be, balanced or otherwise. (It can also show us why there is often nothing more unbalancing than the demand for a balanced view.) We can only be really realistic after we have tried our optimism out. It is not always clear in which areas of our lives it is realistic (or even optimistic) to aspire to the balanced view; or indeed in which parts of our lives the balanced view helps us to get the lives that we want. Balancing acts are entertaining because they are risky, but there are situations in which it is more dangerous to keep your balance than to lose it.

Psychoanalysis has been good at giving us pictures of childhood that we can use in adult life; it shows us that the lives we did and didn't live as children are clues to the lives we want as adults and it also shows us that, beyond a certain point, being a nice person – just like being a nasty person – means being too fearful of one's own nature. It tries to persuade us, for example, that we sometimes get our picture of morality from the child's struggle to be continent. We tend to think of morality now as more to do with self-control than poise, more about holding back than going forward, more about discipline than about tact. Gravity, after all, is about what we have to touch. But it is worth wondering whether we could learn better things about morality from the child learning to walk, say, than from toilet-training. Or whether, as Mill intimates, balance is an analogy we shouldn't pursue. Or indeed whether balance, in any of its many senses, is a necessary good (or, as in, say, gymnastics, should balance be a means but not an end?). When it comes to morality, or the making of decisions, or to walking, what are the alternatives to balance?

What we do when we are off balance tends to be more morally interesting than what we do when we are unbalanced. Children may sometimes love making themselves giddy, but adults hate falling over. We want our judges and our juries to make balanced decisions, but we always need our parents to decide in our favour. Siblings never get the same from their parents; it never balances out, despite the parents' wishes. A lot can hang on what we use balance to do, on when our balancing acts are in order.

When Shylock demands his 'pound of flesh' in the fourth act of *The Merchant of Venice*, and Portia, disguised as a judge, replies in kind, 'Are there balance here to weigh/ The flesh?' we are naturally horrified by the literalness of the question, to which Shylock replies straightforwardly, 'I have them ready.' Running together the scales of the merchant and the scales of justice, Shylock's insistent demand for his 'pound of flesh' from Antonio – 'that phrase,' the critic Marjorie Garber writes, 'that floats so oddly through modern language as if it were only and entirely a figure of speech' – reveals just how unbalanced the balanced view can be (and, indeed, what is at stake in the balancing acts of everyday life: in the making of comparisons and the wreaking of revenge). If balance is not the thing, what is? If a balanced view is not what we seek, what are the alternatives? It is what Hazlitt called the 'hard, impenetrable, dark groundwork of the character of Shylock' that makes us ask these questions, and that makes *The Merchant of Venice* such a disturbing play. On balance; in the words of Antonio, 'Is that anything now?'

Five Short Talks on Excess*

It is very stretchy.

Kay Ryan, 'The Fabric of Life'

I In Excess

Nothing makes people more excessive than talking about excess. We tend to become either extremely disapproving or unusually enthusiastic and excited about the most recently reported celebrity orgy, or managing director's pay rise. No one can be indifferent to binge drinking, or the amount of pornography on the internet; everyone knows someone now who has a so-called 'eating disorder', and everyone knows about the huge numbers of people in the world who are starving. Excess is everywhere now — excesses of wealth and of poverty, of sex and greed, of violence and of religious belief. If the twentieth century was, in the

---

* These were talks for BBC Radio 3 and have been kept in their original form.

title of historian Eric Hobsbawm's book, *The Age of Extremes*, then the twenty-first century looks like being the Age of Excess. When people are being extreme they push things to their limits; when they are being excessive they push things beyond their limits.

I want here to explore our fear and loathing, our fascination and craving for excess in all its forms. And I want to bear in mind something very strange about excess, something best pictured perhaps by the extraordinary consumerism of Western societies, or by the religious and anti-religious fanaticism in contemporary culture; and that is that excess is contagious. Nothing makes people more excessive than talking about excess.

Like a lot of the words we use very easily, 'excess' is older than we imagine. *The Oxford English Dictionary* dates its earliest, most literal meaning of 'the action of going out or forth' to the fifteenth century; 'excess', in its original use, being the opposite of 'access'. And this, too, I think is something we should bear in mind: access, if you like, is the freedom to go in; excess is the freedom to go out. But when we are excessive what are we going out from?

Here, again, the dictionary can help us, and this time into more familiar territory: when we are excessive we 'depart from custom [or] reason', we 'overstep' limits, we go beyond our 'rights'; we are involved in what the dictionary calls 'extravagant violation of law, decency or morality', we are guilty of 'outrageous conduct'. When we are excessive, in whatever way, we depart from what is considered appropriate behaviour; we go out from, we abandon, the version of ourselves we are supposed to be. And where do we get our standards of appropriate behaviour, our pictures of ourselves as we are supposed to be? From the societies we grow up in. Excess, the dictionary reminds us, is not simply the violation of law, decency or morality, it is the '*extravagant* violation of law, decency or morality'. So excess covers a whole gamut of experiences from exaggeration to breaking the law, from boasting to genocide. The anorexic and the suicide bomber, the attention-seeking child and the compulsive gambler, the person who has more money than he needs and the person committed to celibacy are all involved, in their different ways, in extravagant violations of law, decency or morality; even though, of course, they may not see it this way. And this, too, is important when we are thinking about excess: what is excessive to one person may be to another person just an ordinary way of life. The devoutly religious are not, in their own view, over-doing it; terrorists are not, in their view, overreacting to the injustices they feel they have suffered. Indeed, one of the ways of describing many of our personal and political and religious conflicts is that someone is trying to persuade someone else that they are being excessive: excessively cruel, excessively disrespectful, excessively unjust. So we need to remember just how much can hang on our definitions of excess. I want to consider here what might make us feel, in any given situation, that someone is being excessive; and what, when we feel people are being excessive, we want to do about it. Our knee-jerk reaction is often to want to punish them, and often excessively. And yet people usually punish each other when they don't know what else to do; which is why punishment is so often beside the point, an excited failure of imagination. Punishment is despair about the rules, not their enforcement. So it isn't just that excess is contagious, but that other people's excess permits us, or even frees us, to be excessive ourselves. Our reactions to other people's excesses – of violence, of appetite, of belief – are, as we shall see, extremely revealing. 'All truths,' the philosopher Alain Badiou writes, 'are woven from extreme consequences.' There are also truths woven from excessive consequences.

But perhaps one thing we shouldn't lose sight of is just how reassuring the whole idea of excess can be; when we are not permitted to take excess baggage on the plane it is because somebody is keeping an eye on our safety, somebody knows how much the plane can take. In other words, what is reassuring about the idea of excess – about our being able to think that someone is being excessive – is that it implies that we know our limits, that we have a sure sense of the proper way to behave, that we know what is appropriate and right. Every time we have the moralistic version of the excess experience – the righteous indignation, or rage, or grief about the transgressions of other people – we relocate ourselves, firmly and safely, within the rules, the protective walls, of our societies. In these moments we are reminded of how the world should be, and that someone who knows the rules and can enforce them is looking after us. The child who has a tantrum is trying to find out if his parents are robust, whether they can withstand his hatred and rage and frustration. In this instance excessive behaviour is an opportunity for the parents to remind themselves, or for society to remind itself, of established rules and regulations. It reassures us to see that we clearly know what the rules are because we are outraged when they are broken.

If we are so good at spotting excessive behaviour when we see it – excessive eating, excessive sex, excessive shopping, the excessive beliefs of religious fanatics – then we must know, or think we know, what just the right amount of these things is. If we can recognize greed when we see it, we must know how people should eat; if we can be appalled by the sexual excesses reported in the tabloids, we must know what kind of sex people should be having, and how often they should be having it; if we are full of righteous indignation about people we think of as 'religious fanatics', we must surely have very strong ideas about how much people should believe things, about what people should believe in and what their beliefs should drive them to do. But what is the right amount of belief? How do we know when someone's grief is excessive? Perhaps when it makes us feel something more excessive than we would like to feel?

There is an obvious irony here: many of the things that matter most to us – like love, or grief, or appetite, or violence, or political and religious belief – cannot be measured; and yet one of the things we are most alert to, one of the things we speak about with the most passionate conviction, is when we feel these things have become excessive. It is as if we have our own internal measure of these things that can't be quantified; and this internal measure is one of the most important things about us. How could we live without a sense of what is excessive? Indeed, as I have said, is it not striking how excessive we can be in our reactions to other people's excesses? Nothing makes us more excessive than excess; nothing makes us more disapproving, disgusted, punitive – not to mention fascinated, exhilarated and amazed – than other people's extravagant appetite for food, or alcohol, or money, or drugs, or violence; nothing makes us more frightened, more furious, more despairing than other people's extreme commitment to political ideals or religious beliefs. It is, one should notice, almost always other people who are being excessive in their belief, not oneself. 'One is never, in any way whatever, overwhelmed by another person's excesses,' the French psychoanalyst Jacques Lacan once said, 'one is only and always overwhelmed because their excesses happen to coincide with your own.' From a psychoanalytic point of view other people's excesses disturb us, get us worked up, because they reveal something important to us about ourselves; about our own fears and longings. Indeed, other people's excesses might reveal to us, at its most minimal, that we are, or have become, the excessive animals; the animals for whom excessive behaviour is the rule rather than the exception (there are laws of human nature, but not for us). You only have to read the newspapers to realize that this is a plausible possibility. Our excesses may be in excess of our capacity to understand and to regulate. And if we have become the excessive animals we may have to do more than merely aspire not to be.

When Lacan suggests that we are only overwhelmed by other people's excesses because they are the same as our own he is not simply saying, for example, that our horror about drug addiction means that we are secretly tempted or prone to become drug addicts; but that drug addiction may be a picture, say, of how fearful we might be generally of our own dependence, how terrified we are of becoming enslaved to the people we need. And drug addiction can also be a picture of how tempted we are to try to become everything that the person we love needs; to become, in a way, their drug of choice. In other words, Lacan's point is that our reaction to other people's excesses is an important clue to something vital about ourselves; our reflex response to other people's excessive behaviour — the thrill of righteous indignation, the moral superiority of our disgust – is more complex and more interesting than it at first seems. If other people's excesses reveal the bigot in us, they also reveal how intriguing and subtle the bigot is. There is nothing more telling, nothing more revealing of one's own character and history and taste, than one's reaction to other people's excesses. Tell me which kinds of excess fascinate you, tell me which kinds of excess appal you, and I will tell you who you are. This would be one, excessive, way of putting it. Or one could more sensibly say: notice which excesses you are drawn to (and there is, of course, an excess of excesses to choose from now – road rage, fundamentalism, self-improvement, shopping), the ones you can't stop complaining about, the ones that make you speak out, or the ones that just give you some kind of secret, perhaps slightly embarrassing pleasure, and try to work out what about them is so compelling.

Excessive behaviour, it seems obvious to say, attracts our attention; what is perhaps less obvious is why it should do so. We are excessively interested in the excessive behaviour that interests us; and to be excessively interested is to be more interested than we would like to be. So even though it would be silly to say that our reaction to other people's excesses is the key to our nature – because there is no key to our nature – it is true to say, I think, that our reactions to other people's excesses reveal to us what our conflicts are. I don't want to be a drug addict, but I do want to be free to need someone; and I don't want to lose my life when I do need them. I don't want to be a suicide bomber, but I may want to have something in my life that is so important to me that I would risk my life for it; or I may simply want to be aggressive enough to be able to protect the people I love. Or I may even want to have the courage of my despair. The excesses of other people, and of ourselves, can make us think, rather than merely react. Indeed, something as powerful as excess might – if we can suspend our fear – allow us to have thoughts we have never had before. After all, inspiration, falling in love, conversion experiences, a sense of injustice – the most radical transformations that can occur in a life – are traditionally overwhelming, excessive experiences. Even though we often want to get over them, to get back to normal as quickly as possible. 'For the doctrine of conversion,' the Victorian classicist Benjamin Jowett wrote, 'the moralist substitutes the theory of habit.' And nothing, of course, is more excessive than a habit.

So perhaps when the poet William Blake wrote in his 'Proverbs of Hell' that 'The road of excess leads to the Palace of Wisdom' he wasn't joking? We don't tend to look to anorexics or gluttons, to the extravagantly rich or the promiscuous, for wisdom; we don't think of drug addicts or mass murderers as necessarily enlightened. So perhaps Blake was being ironic; they are, after all, 'Proverbs of Hell'. Perhaps the road of excess, through the very disillusionments it produces, is a source of wisdom; that it is not the alcoholic but the recovering alcoholic who has something to tell us. Perhaps as part of growing up we *need* to be excessive – to try to break all the rules just to be able to find out what, if anything, the rules are made of, and why they matter. Perhaps only the road of excess can teach us when enough is enough. (And perhaps 'perhaps' – like all our cherished rhetoric of self-doubt – is one way we temper our excesses in language.) As Blake says, in another of his proverbs, 'You never know what is enough unless you know what is more than enough.' Either certain kinds of excess are not simply good for us, but essential to our well-being; or we need to go through excessive experiences to discover what they can't do for us, to discover just how much of something we really need. But what is a Palace of Wisdom? And why would that be a good place to go to?

II Enough is Enough

When the novelist Thomas Mann was a child his father contrived an experiment to teach him and his siblings a lesson about appetite. 'Our father assured us,' Mann writes, 'that once in our lives we could eat as many cream puffs ... and cream rolls at the pastry shop as we wanted. He led us into a sweet-smelling Paradise, and let the dream become reality – and we were amazed how quickly we reached the limit of our desire, which we had believed to be infinite.' Here the road of excess does lead to the Palace of Wisdom; what the young Thomas Mann discovers, reassuringly, is that his appetite has a natural limit; in anticipation his youthful hunger may be excessive, but when it comes to it he is amazed how quickly, as he puts it, 'we reached the limit of our desire'. We only need to experiment with our greed to discover that it is only in our fantasies that we are excessive; in reality our appetite is sensible; is, as we like to say, self-regulating. We know when we have had enough.

But it is, of course, still worth wondering why, in our fantasy lives, we tend to be so excessive; why, at least in fantasy, excessive appetite and its satisfaction is so appealing to us. When the singer Neil Diamond was asked how he felt about being rich, he said, 'You can't have two lunches.' It would be a relief to believe that excess is just something we imagine; that if we were very rich, if we could eat as much as we liked, we would discover just how reasonable we really are.

You may not be able to have two lunches, but you can have one very long lunch; and children, as we know, given half a chance, can all too easily make themselves sick by eating, say, too much chocolate. Clearly we would like to believe that we are not by nature excessive creatures; that excess is a sign of something being wrong. Excessive appetite, we might say, is a symptom. And Thomas Mann gives us a clue about what it might be a symptom of in the way he tells his story. 'Our father assured us,' he wrote, 'that once in our lives we could eat as many cream puffs ... as we wanted'; but why only once? No reliable scientific experiment is performed only once. It is as though the father knew that once would be enough. Perhaps the experiment was a set-up to prove the father's authority – or perhaps Mann was suggesting in this story that there is only one thing more excessive than appetite, at least for a child, and that is his excessive belief in his father's authority. What the experiment proved was how much the children wanted to be what their father wanted them to be; it proved that they were not really greedy but well-behaved. History would prove that in Thomas Mann's Germany it was the appetite for authority that was excessive; people would do literally anything for their Fatherland, for their Führer.

We might say, then, that excessive behaviour reveals a failure of authority; that only children with weak parents are excessive. From a psychoanalytic point of view we might even say – in support of the law-and-order lobby – that when young people are being excessive they are unconsciously – without realizing it – trying to find strong, containing parents. Unruly adolescents, for example, can be thought of as needing to find out just how reliable, just how robust and impressive, the authorities really are. And even though this is an often useful account – that children are only as powerful as their parents let them be, and that there is nothing the child is more frightened of than being too powerful – there is something in this view that we need to notice. Excess, as I have argued, is contagious. We always meet one kind of excess with another. In this case an excessive belief in authority is taken to be the cure for excesses of appetite. At its crudest this translates as: greed is simply a need for authority, and the greedy need to be intimidated or blackmailed. In this cartoon the authorities say: if you curb, or even renounce, the excesses of your appetite, we will love and protect you, and even, in some religions, reward you with eternal life. But if you don't, we won't. These are desperate measures. We seem to be the only animals for whom appetite is excessive, the only animals who eat more than they need, and we have settled into this view. Most of us live now as if we are more or less reconciled to the fact that too many people are starving while too many people are eating too much.

The excesses in our world may be shocking, but we adapt to them remarkably well. We take excess for granted now, and are horrified by it at the same time. (Or, rather, we need to distinguish between the excesses we can too readily adapt to, and those we cannot.) We need to consider the possibility that we are addicted to the picture of ourselves as the excessive animals, excessively impressed by it. Is there more to say than that we are born greedy and need, one way or another, to learn to control ourselves? Clearly discipline, control and punishment matter so much to us because we see ourselves as excessive (and because, of course, they give us so much insidious pleasure); but if the road of excess leads to the Palace of Wisdom, this is pretty thin wisdom – that we are born out of control, born too hungry, and need to pull ourselves together; that life is about learning to be sufficiently contained. That the very thing our survival depends upon – our appetite – is the one thing that is too much for us. We need to go back to a beginning – not *the* beginning, but *a* beginning – and ask some simple questions.

Why, if we wanted something, if we loved something – like cream cakes, or particular people – would we want too much of it? And, by the same token, why, if we wanted something, if we loved something, would we want too little of it? All these dilemmas, unsurprisingly, start in childhood. At the very start of our lives our mothers, or the people who care for us, are food, and everything associated with food — comfort, safety, reassurance, excitement: a mother feeding a child is a picture of someone understanding someone else's need and, ideally, of someone wanting to satisfy someone. Being fed relieves one's suffering, and meets one's excitement. In most so-called ordinary development most mothers and babies find a way through to this good experience. Greed, what we think of as excessive appetite, mostly turns up in older children; and all children, as they grow up, develop conflicts about eating. In this sense it is normal for children to have 'issues' about eating, and these issues are always about too much and too little. Growing up is the discovery of one's appetite; and it is one's appetite that links one to other people.

So, to return to our questions: why, from a psychoanalytic point of view, if we wanted something, if we loved something — a mother or a cream cake — why would we want too much of it? Well, we might fear losing it and never having it again, so we might believe that we need to take it all and hoard it for ever; that because it could go away, or run out, or someone else could take it, we had better get as much as we can. Or we may become greedy because what we are getting is not quite what we want: it's failing to satisfy me so I begin to believe that more is better, that if one cream cake isn't doing the trick, three will, when in fact it isn't a cream cake that I really want.

Or I might become greedy out of envy: I realize that the cakes and the mother that I love don't actually belong to me, but I depend upon them being available; and because I can't bear the fact that I actually depend upon them I would rather destroy them with my greed. There is always a magical belief that by destroying the thing that we love we destroy our need for it. And, finally, greed is a way of avoiding making choices: if I have everything I don't have to choose what I want. And choosing what I want means giving up some pleasures for other pleasures.

We are greedy, then, because we fear losing what we need; because we fear that it isn't the right thing; because we fear depending on something that doesn't belong to us; and because we fear making choices. When we are greedy, the psychoanalyst Harold Boris writes, we are in a state of mind in which we 'wish and hope to have everything all the time'; greed 'wants everything, nothing less will do', and so 'it cannot be satisfied'. Appetite, he explains in a useful distinction, 'is inherently satisfiable. It goes after what it wants and yet is receptive to what it gets. It makes do, not letting ... the better stand in the way of the good ... Greed ... cannot be satisfied.' So the excess of appetite we call greed is actually a form of despair. Greed turns up when we lose faith in our appetites, when what we need is not available. In this view it is not that appetite is excessive; it is that our fear of frustration is excessive. Excess is a sign of frustration; we are only

excessive wherever there is a frustration we are unaware of, and a fear we cannot bear. An addiction is
an unformulated frustration.

And so why, if we wanted or loved something,
would we want too little of it? What would make us
become either literally, or metaphorically, anorexic?
What would make us refuse the very things that sustain us? I remember asking a nine-year-old child in
therapy why he would never, as his mother put it,
'finish his plate'. He said, quite sensibly, 'If I finish it
there won't be any left,' and then he paused and added,
'I'll be hungry for ever.' I said, 'So eating is like killing Mummy,' and he grinned and said, 'Killing her
for ever.' For this boy, eating enough was eating too
much; and eating too much was linked in his mind
with losing his mother. He always asked his mother
to keep the food he left 'for tomorrow'.

As it turns out, we eat too little for the same reasons
that we eat too much. The child, the psychoanalyst
D. W. Winnicott writes, can 'use doubt about food
to hide doubt about love'; doubt about love is doubt
about resources. And it would make sense that the
child who has some doubt about whether what he
needs is available – which is, of course, every child to
some extent – will try to wean himself off his needs,
will try to make himself self-sufficient, independent
of other people. But once again excess – here, excessive deprivation – is born of mortal fear. Excesses
of appetite are self-cures for feelings of helplessness.

And if this is true, or at least sometimes true, it means that when we are punishing people for their excesses, we are punishing them for their helplessness. Perhaps it is our excessive helplessness, our relative power-lessness faced with the difficulties of living, that we are trying to abolish? Punishing people, after all, can make us feel excessively powerful. But the one thing we tend not to notice about punishment is how rarely it works.

What we learn, then, from the road of excess, is about our frustration, and about how difficult it can be for us to locate what it is that we do need; and consumer capitalism has taught us to be phobic of frustration. Whenever we have too much, it is because there is too little of what we need; whenever we have too little it is because there is too much of what we don't need. We are what we think of as excessively hungry when we have waited too long to eat, or when what we have eaten hasn't satisfied us. Excess, in other words, is always linked to some kind of deprivation. So it may not be certain kinds of excessive behaviour we hate, whether we express this as a terror of our children becoming anorexic, or a preju-dice against fat people, or disgust that there are celebrity chefs in a world of starving people; it may be that we hate excessive behaviour because it reminds us of our own and other people's deprivations. That the bad news which greed brings us is not that we are the insatiable animals who need to control ourselves, but that we are the frustrated animals who can't easily identify what we need, and who are terrified of the experience of frustration. Excessive behaviour is the best way we have come up with so far for dealing with frustration: or, rather, excessive behaviour gives us the illusion that we have got rid of our frustration, that we have forgotten that we were ever frustrated.

It would be comforting to think that if we could only locate our real needs and get them met we would no longer need to be the animals that we are: excessive in our appetites, and excessive in our refusals of appetite. And yet it seems more likely that we are always going to have only a limited capacity to recognize our needs; and that there will always be a scarcity of resources (and, of course, when we are being greedy we can forget that there is not unlimited food). It is clearly good for us to try to get a better sense of what our needs might be, and good for us to be as inventive as we can be to increase our resources. But the other thing that might be true is that we have become excessively frightened of feeling frustrated; why else do people in affluent countries eat so much more than they need – indeed, make a cult of eating? Is it because we have become, have been encouraged to be, phobic of frustration? As though satisfaction is more enlivening, more interesting, more revealing than frustration. We can only be truly satisfied if we are truly frustrated. Excesses of appetite are the ways we conceal from ourselves what we hunger for. As Kafka's 'A Hunger Artist' — the man in the story of that name, who does performance-fasting for a living — replies when asked why he has devoted his life to starving himself in public; he couldn't help doing it, he says, 'because I couldn't find the food I liked. If I had found it, believe me, I should have made no fuss and stuffed myself like you and everyone else.' But what if satisfaction is rather more elusive than this suggests, or indeed that our pictures of satisfaction are radically misleading and distract us from our wanting? If sex, for example, didn't have to satisfy us it might give us more pleasure.

III Sex Mad

One of the more interesting mysteries about growing up is how we get from being creatures with an appetite for food to creatures with an appetite for sex. They are, we might say, two stages in the quest for love, or at least for some sort of satisfaction; and from a Darwinian point of view they are the preconditions of our existence: the first project is survival, the second project is reproduction. And yet one of the striking things about human sexuality is just how apparently self-destructive it can be, and how much of it, to all intents and purposes, doesn't seem to be in the service of reproduction at all. Whereas other animals' sexuality is entirely governed by a reproductive cycle, ours is not. And nothing seems to destabilize us more – nothing seems to make our lives more difficult from adolescence onwards – than our sexual desire. 'It is terrible to desire and not possess, and terrible to possess and not desire,' the poet W. B. Yeats wrote. Falling in love and falling in lust irredeemably exposes just how excessive we can be. The whole of Western literature is about what people do for love; for love of something or someone. For love of love.

But what is most striking, and begins with puberty, is how sexuality makes fantasizers of us all; and whether the fantasies are pornographic or romantic, intensely exciting or mildly distracting, they are very often excessive in the satisfactions that they promise. Why, again, in our fantasy lives do we tend to be so excessive, even if in so-called reality we are more measured, rather better behaved? A simple answer would be that in our fantasies – in what D. H. Lawrence called our 'sex in the head' – we can have things exactly as we want them. That when our fantasies are excessively satisfying there is no frustration in them; they reveal, in other words, a fear of frustration. And yet, of course, we quite literally can't bear hunger beyond a certain point; and while we may despair without sexual satisfaction, we can survive. One of the differences between hunger and sexual appetite is that we all began with somebody appointed, as it were, to feed us; we do not, in any sense, begin with someone appointed to have sex with us. If we have been lucky, and had good-enough early care from our parents – if, that is to say, they have been sufficiently reliable and available – we will discover, in adolescence, that the objects of sexual desire, the people and the experiences we want, are surprisingly elusive. Mostly, when we cried with hunger we were fed. When we desire someone, when we long for someone sexually, as adults, it is never that simple. The excesses of fantasy – the fundamentalism of fantasy – keep us hopeful in a very uncertain world.

When it comes to sexuality, once again, excess is the sign of the fear of scarcity, a way of keeping our spirits up. But there are, of course, drawbacks to just how satisfying, just how pleasurable, sexual and romantic fantasies can be. Because fantasy formulates the mismatch between what we want and what is there. As Anna Freud once famously said, 'In our dreams we can have our eggs cooked exactly how we want them, but we can't eat them.' So satisfying are our fantasies that they can become a refuge, a retreat from reality; if real sexual relations are too difficult – too frustrating, too pleasurable – in our fantasies we can have our relationships cooked exactly as we want them. Our fantasies, in other words, may reveal that we are not excessively sexual, but excessively frightened of other people. That our fantasies at once formulate our desires – often in disguised form – and render them reassuringly impossible to realize. It is not that reality is disappointing, but that fantasies, in their very excess, are unrealistic.

'Our desire,' Freud wrote, 'is always in excess of the object's capacity to satisfy it.' We always want more than we can have; but we are more inclined to blame the world for letting us down than to notice just how unrealistic our desires are. But why would our desire be excessive? One reason might be that our disappointment keeps us going; that we keep ourselves desiring by hoping for a satisfaction that will never come; or that we must ensure will never come. Because we are frustrated we keep on wanting. And this does make sense; wanting more means never giving up, as though one of the temptations we are always warding off is giving up; the very excesses of our sexual desire, our insistent quest for love and satisfaction, keeps this hopelessness at bay. Or perhaps, as Freud among many others also suggests, we are simply excessively, insistently, unavoidably sexually-driven creatures. Our desire for love and sex is insatiable. It's not the problem, it's the point.

It is as though we have two choices: either we think that some people quite explicitly, or all people rather more secretly, are obsessed by sex; or we think, as excess tends to make us think, that sexual excess is a symptom of something. What, we can ask, are people who are having too much sex, having too much of? Or, what are people who want too much sex – who are, as we say now, in the Age of Diagnosis, sex addicts – avoiding? Does too much sex mean too little so-called relationship? Are sex addicts frightened of what we call intimacy? When the Christian Right described AIDS as God's punishment of homosexuals the implication was not only that they were being punished for being gay, but that they were also being punished because being gay supposedly meant having too much sex. Beyond a certain point, beyond a certain amount – though it is always unspecified – too much sex, one way or another, is bad. In our world of weights and measures, too much of one thing is always assumed to be too little of something else; too little of something else that is better.

Too much sex, broadly speaking, means too little concern for other people. It means sex that harms people who haven't consented to being harmed. And yet too much sex can also mean more sex than I am having and would like to have. When it comes to the excesses of sexuality we can't always tell whether our morality is a cover story for our envy, or simply a rationalization of our fear; we would like to be that excited, that promiscuous, that abandoned, but it is too much of a risk for us. The two 'Proverbs of Hell' that follow Blake's 'The road of excess leads to the Palace of Wisdom' are: 'Prudence is a rich, ugly old maid courted by Incapacity' and 'He who desires but acts not, breeds pestilence.' We don't, on the whole, tend to envy other people's appetite for food, but other people's appetite for sex — especially in a society in which sex represents health, vitality and youth — gets to us. Nothing makes people more excessive than talking about excess. People are even more excessive when they talk about sexual excesses. The person who haunts us is the person who is having more pleasure than us. Our tantalizing double.

We have a set of equations that we have been educated to live by: a good sexual appetite equals aliveness, but because sex can be excessively pleasurable and excessively frustrating we fear it, so sex also equals inhibition (we never feel quite as free sexually as we could be); but a good sexual appetite also brings with it the possibility of promiscuity, of infidelity and betrayal, and all the suffering involved, so sex also equals havoc and torment. So a freer sexuality equals a fuller, more uninhibited life, but by the same token, a life in which more harm is done. The excesses of our sexuality, as everyone knows, bring with them an excess of what we have learned to call problems. It is, as we say, all too much. We can affect a breeziness about sexuality − a sex-is-fun blitheness − but we take these positions only because we know how much is at stake. 'There is no sex without love or its refusal,' the writer Paul Goodman once said. When we speak of what we think of as excessive sexualities we either become earnestly moralistic or overly casual. It is indeed worth noting that excesses − and excessive sexual behaviours are a good example of this − tend to polarize people, to narrow people's minds. As if we don't quite have the equipment, the vocabulary, for dealing with our own excesses; as though language itself is not suited to excess, is not made for it. Our attitudes to these extremes of sexuality tend towards the moralistically permissive, or the moralistically prohibitive − both equally dogmatic positions. Perhaps we have to find a way of resisting being excessive when we talk about excess; or of being excessive in more intriguing ways. And sex might be a good place to start.

'The construction of erotic excitement,' the way in which each of us gets sexually excited, the psychoanalyst Robert Stoller writes, 'is every bit as subtle,

complex, inspired, profound, tidal, fascinating, awesome, problematic, unconscious-soaked, and genius-
haunted as the creation of dreams or art.' This, one
might feel, is excessive, but it is the kind of excess that
opens up the conversation rather than closes it down,
as the extreme moral positions do. It says, at its most
minimal, that sexual excitement – sexual desire and its
enactment – is far more interesting, far more complex,
and far more revealing than we might have imagined.
By comparing our erotic lives to works of art, Stoller
is reminding us that there may not be quite as much
difference as we think between a vocation, a passion
and an obsession; all are forms of excess, but we don't
call artists art addicts, or religious people God addicts.
In other words, the excesses of our sexuality, so enthu-
siastically evoked by Stoller, may be more akin to more
culturally sanctioned, more highly valued kinds of
cultural activity than we would like to imagine. Stoller
suggests that we should talk about people's erotic life
more as art critics talk about art; and what he means
by this is that we should be working out what our sexuality may be about, and what the experience is like –
what it aspires to tell us about ourselves and others
– rather than judging it pre-emptively. Excess makes
us judge things before we find out what they are.

It is very common these days for men to come for
psychoanalytic treatment with problems of commitment. 'Commitment' itself, of course, has an interesting double meaning; a commitment is both an order

to send someone to prison or to a mental hospital, and
it is also an obligation willingly undertaken. People
are committed to their partners, and can be committed to hospital. These men with so-called commitment problems are either more promiscuous than
they want to be, or more celibate than they want to
be. But what do the excessive forms that their sexuality has taken tell them if we drop the prevailing
assumption that they are simply more Men Behaving
Badly? The psychoanalyst has a simple choice faced
with these excesses: he can either try to find a way,
with all the techniques and intuitions at his disposal,
to get the man to behave better. And if he takes this
option he must, of course, already know what it
would be for such a man to be better; and in all likeli-
hood this would be conformity with one of the several cultural norms available. If the treatment works
the man will be more considerate, less hurtful, more
responsible and concerned about the meanings and
the consequences of his actions. Even though, as
Blake wrote, 'He who desires but acts not, breeds
pestilence,' the man may discover that acting on too
many of his desires also breeds pestilence. In a certain
sense, of course, this is a caricature; but in this version the cure for excessive promiscuity or excessive
celibacy could be described as excessive conformity.
This man might become loveable to those people
who share this morality, this view of what relations
between the sexes should consist of. What could an

alternative option be? If we don't regulate, discipline or punish sexual excesses, what are we going to do? And we have to answer this question mindful of the fact that just wanting to explore and understand excessive, bad behaviour can be a kind of complicity. An excess of understanding and curiosity and empathy might just be more of the problem.

You will notice that in the supposed cure of these sexual excesses – as in the disciplining and the punishing of them – there is no news; the excesses of these men's sexuality brings nothing new to the Palace of Wisdom. Even the analyst intent on understanding is likely to be able to understand only those things he already knows. 'Literature,' Ezra Pound said – though he could have been speaking of all the arts – 'is news that stays news.' If erotic life is seen as a work of art, then the alternative to reassuring conformity is to have an ear for the new, for the surprising, for the unexpected. We don't have relationships to get our needs met, we have relationships to discover what our needs might be. Good descriptions of our sexuality allow for their being news about it. You can't be a know-all about sex. Our often unconscious assumptions about sexuality stop us having new thoughts about it.

Perhaps our excessive sexualities – and the excesses in our so-called normal sexualities – are showing us something we haven't already thought about ourselves. When we are sexually excessive we are like people who have to shout, people who have to insist, people who have to force themselves on our attention because no one – including ourselves – has been able to hear what they are saying (the speaker one tends not to listen to is oneself). We are pushy only when we assume people won't cooperate, won't get what we are on about. Our sexual excesses reveal just how enigmatic our erotic lives really are – and how much we use our sexuality to say other things about ourselves. When we talk of our sexuality as being excessive we should be asking, excessive compared to what? Compared to our fairness, compared to our reasonableness, compared to our wish to know ourselves? The question may not be: how can we be less excessive? but which of our excesses brings us the life we want? And, of course, how are we going to find this out?

IV On Being Too Much for Ourselves

It is not unusual for us to feel that life is too much for us. And it is not unusual to feel that we really should be up to it; that there may be too much to cope with – too many demands – but that we should have the wherewithal to deal with it. Faced with the stresses and strains of everyday life it is easy now for people to feel that they are failing; and what they are failing at, one way or another, is managing the ordinary excesses that we are all beset by: too much frustration, too much bad feeling, too little love, too little success, and so on. One of the things people most frequently say in psychoanalysis is, 'Perhaps I am overreacting, but . . .'; and one of the commonest complaints today is about feeling too much or feeling too little. I want to suggest that we are simply too much for ourselves, but that this too-muchness is telling us something important. I want to begin with a simple proposition, and see where it takes us. My proposition is that it is impossible to overreact. That when we call our reactions overreactions what we mean is just that they are stronger than we would like them to be. In other words, we sometimes call ourselves and other people excessive as a way of invalidating or tempering the truths we tell ourselves or that other people tell us. It is impossible to overreact.

One of Freud's now famous examples of the over-
reaction is the Freudian slip, when we say more than
we intend. A person I was seeing in psychoanalysis
once said to me, 'Don't you think Fraud is rather overrated'; he had of course meant to say 'Freud', and he
blushed. Embarrassment, blushing, is of course a sign
of excess, the excessive bodily reaction to excessive
self-exposure. In that moment he had said both what
he wanted to say, and rather more than he wanted to
say. When we make Freudian slips we try to cover our
tracks by claiming that we have said more than we
mean, when in fact we have meant more than we had
wanted to say. This man also thought that Freud was a
fraud, and that, of course, is something worth considering; as is the idea that fraud is overrated. When we
make Freudian slips we may feel like we are saying too
much, but we may be saying just the right amount;
adding things to the conversation that are worth talking about and trying out. We can't decide not to make
Freudian slips; but even when we use ordinary language intentionally, we often say more than we intend.
If I say to you that I am a great admirer of your work,
I am telling you about my greatness as well as yours;
when I say, 'See you tomorrow,' I am assuming I know
what isn't going to happen in the interim. Our language, without which we couldn't imagine our lives,
is too much for us in the sense that it can surprise us:
we hear in it – and we say in it – more than we intend
to. And more than we attend to.

We spend our earliest years looking and hearing and touching and smelling before we can speak; language comes to us, in a sense, quite late in the day. And these so-called early years are, to put it mildly, years of intense feeling. What the critic Lee Edelman calls, in a usefully provocative phrase, 'the fascist face of the baby' captures something of the sheer power of the child's feelings, and their effect on the people around them. If the cry of a crying baby wasn't, in some sense, too much for us — something we have to respond to, something we need to stop, if possible — the baby wouldn't survive. And all parents at some time feel overwhelmed by their children; feel that their children ask more of them than they can provide. One of the most difficult things about being a parent is that you have to bear the fact that you have to frustrate your child, have to make your child suffer more than he wants to: and this means every parent has to bear being hated by their children, and hatred between parents and children always feels excessive.

We have all had the experience, as children, of being too much for someone; of making someone feel things that they didn't want to feel. Before you have children, the novelist Fay Weldon once said, you can believe you are a nice person: after you have children you understand how wars start. Everyone starts with the experience of being too much for someone else; not only with that experience, but with that experience somewhere in the mix of who one is.

Before we acquire the limiting and limited excesses of language we have lived with the excesses of need. If, even only occasionally as a child, you are too much for your parents – which then means you are too much for yourself – what can you do?

We call someone's behaviour excessive when it does harm that seems unnecessary to us, or when it inflicts more suffering than we think it should. The child who experiences himself as being too much for his parents – all children to some extent – experiences himself as in some way harming them. And as the child's survival depends upon his parents, or those who look after him, this puts him in mortal danger. For this reason alone it is very difficult for the child – and for the adult that he will become – to think of his too-muchness as anything other than a problem. And yet, of course, parents are there to absorb, and be absorbed in, their children's excesses (and vice versa). Indeed, people know that they are in a relationship when they become a problem to each other (or, to put it slightly differently, if you want to have a relation-ship with someone you have to become a problem for them). How could being too much for other people and for oneself be anything other than something one needs to get over? How can making the people you love suffer be, in any sense, a good thing? We can begin to make some sense of this, perhaps, by asking a simple question: why do people exaggerate?

If you fear not being listened to, if you assume

that you are easily forgotten or can't find a place in other people's minds, you are going to have to do something extreme to hold their attention. I am more likely to get a seat on the bus if I say I have a heart condition than if I say I don't like standing up. Exaggeration is an attempt to capture someone else's imagination, to get a hearing. People are histrionic to get people thinking about them. We are excessive when something about ourselves needs to be recognized and we need other people to help us work out what it is. We are too much for ourselves because there is far more to us – we feel more – than we can manage. People didn't overreact to the death of Diana; through the death of Diana they recognized just how much grief they were bearing, how much loss they had suffered in their lives, how they felt about the fate of young women in our culture. Indeed, grief, rather like sexuality, reminds us just how much we are too much for ourselves, how intense our loves and longings really are. How would we know, who could tell us, whether we were overreacting to someone's death, or, indeed, when our grieving is excessive and should come to an end?

We are too much for ourselves – in our hungers and our desires, in our griefs and our commitments, in our loves and our hates – because we are unable to include so much of what we feel in the picture we have of ourselves. The whole idea of ourselves as excessive exposes how determined we are to have the

wrong picture of what we are like, of how fanat-
ically ignorant we are about ourselves. We describe
people as excessively violent not when they are being
more violent than they really are, or should be, but
because they are being more violent than we want
them to be. They are showing us what people are
capable of: we may want to think that people who
torture others, people who are committed to ethnic
cleansing, people who will kill themselves and others
for their beliefs, are the exceptions that prove the
rule; but actually they reveal to us what certain
people in certain situations, certain predicaments,
want to do. Excessive behaviour tells us more than
we want to hear about who we are, about what we
want to say to each other, and what we might be
capable of. And adolescence – when children begin
to have the physical capacity to murder and conceive
– is our more conscious initiation into those very
excesses that make us who we are; and, of course,
who we might become. Adolescents are excessive
compared with the children they once were and the
adults they are supposed to become. But adolescence,
at least for modern people, seems to be peculiarly
difficult to grow out of. Indeed, one of the biggest
problems that adolescents now have is that the adults
often envy them; and what contemporary adults
tend to envy about adolescents is their excessive
behaviour. The contemporary idealization of adolescence is telling us something about how we manage

our complicated feelings about being too much for ourselves.

We secretly believe adolescents are having more fun, more pleasure, more passionate intensity than we are; and more publicly we talk about how they need to be disciplined. We talk about stamping out knife crimes, but not about how frightened someone might be if they feel they need to carry a knife, nor indeed about how exhilarating and potent a young person might feel carrying a knife. We talk about fear of teenage pregnancy, but not of the intense excitements of discovering sex and being able to experiment with it. Nor do we talk much about the fear and confusion and grief that sexuality brings in its wake because it is so pleasurable, or not pleasurable enough; because it is such an essential part of who we happen to be. With adolescence there is always what the adults think of as excessive behaviour around: excessive isolation, excessive gregariousness, excessive moodiness, too much drink and too many drugs. The adolescent, in other words, tends to meet excess with excess: excessive boredom is cured by excessive excitement, excessive despair is cured by excessive idealism, excessive uncertainty is cured by excessive conviction. But then how do you start to look after yourself after you have been looked after for so long? Human beings, after all, are excessively dependent animals, relying on their parents far longer than any other mammal. And what do you do when you are quite patently more than your parents can cope with, when you (and they) finally cannot avoid the fact that you are too much for them? If, in adolescence, the road of excess leads to the Palace of Wisdom, then the palace of wisdom must be adulthood.

Adolescents are not overreacting to puberty and the world they find themselves in, any more than the parents of adolescents are overreacting in their extremes of rage and delight and despair. Adolescents, and their parents who were once adolescents, are simply experiencing two kinds of helplessness, the helplessness born of experience, and the helplessness born of lack of experience. The adolescents are too much for their parents, and too much for themselves. Parents are just people who have spent more time being too much for themselves. Because adults, of course, are not less excessive in their behaviour than adolescents. Concentration camps were not run by adolescents; adolescents are not mostly alcoholics or millionaires, because they haven't had the time. Excessive behaviour, in other words, is not so much something we grow out of as something we grow into.

We seem only to overreact to the most ordinary things in the world: birth and death, hunger and sex, love and loss, and, of course, ageing. The more we think about the road of excess – of just how excessively excessive we are as animals – the question becomes not, why are we so excessive? but how could we not be, given what we have to deal with?

Perhaps 'excess' is a word we use to reassure ourselves that we can be something other than excessive. If we start off by being, at least some of the time, too much for other people, and become, in adolescence, definitively too much for other people, so much so that we have to leave them, and then become adults who are unavoidably too much for ourselves, what is to be done? Well, one thing that can be done is to find someone we are not too much for, and this, when it isn't an institution or a leader, sometimes has to be a god.

V Believe It or Not

After Adam and Eve have eaten the fateful apple we find them, as Milton writes in *Paradise Lost*, 'bewailing their excess'. By calling the Fall an excess Milton means that it was both a transgression – the breaking of an absolute rule – and an act of greed: by eating the apple they were quite literally, in God's view, eating more than they needed to. Perhaps this is what Blake was alluding to when he writes, in his 'Proverbs of Hell', that 'The road of excess leads to the Palace of Wisdom.' Through their excess Adam and Eve discovered something essential about their own nature that was, perhaps, more than they had wanted to know; that they were, unlike the other animals in the garden, transgressive creatures. Through their excess they discovered much more about themselves and about God; they found out what He does when you break His rules, and they found out that they could indeed break His rules; they realized how free they were, and what kind of Creator their God was. Their only hope after the Fall, they are told by the archangel Michael, is to 'well observe/ The rule of not too much'; they must, from now onwards, seek 'due nourishment, not gluttonous delight'. In a sense it is a simple story: what we must learn from our excesses is the rule of not too much; but Milton gives us pause by opposing sober and sensible 'due nourishment' to the rather more enticing pleasures of 'gluttonous delight'. Do we want to be measured or daring, good and sensible or delighted and excited? In a recent survey a group of old people were asked if they had any regrets about their lives, and the majority of them said they regretted that they had been so virtuous.

We can't talk about religion without talking about excess; which doesn't mean, of course, that everyone who is religious is a fanatic. But it does mean that religious beliefs of any significance matter a great deal to those who hold them. Indeed, they will sometimes sacrifice their lives and the lives of other people for them; their relationship to their gods can be the most important thing in their lives. By definition these gods must be more powerful than the people who believe in them; they are often deemed to be both omniscient and omnipotent. So by human standards gods are excessively powerful, though we are more inclined to think of other people's gods as excessive, and of our own as having just the right amount of power. Once you begin to imply, as Milton sometimes does in *Paradise Lost*, that God may be excessively punitive, you put yourself in the odd position of judging God. It was originally the function of deities to make the rules, which means that it has been traditionally the function of deities to decide what is excessive. There is something God-like, in other words, about describing someone's behaviour as excessive; God knows an excess when He sees one; indeed, He is preoccupied with, if not actually obsessed by, our excesses. Ordinary life for the religious person has to be led, the philosopher Charles Taylor writes, 'in the light of God's ends, ultimately to the glory of God. This means, of course, that one fulfils God's intentions for life, avoiding sin, debauchery, excesses of all sorts ... it means that one lives for God.' God is the one who is supposed to know what counts as excessive, and what the punishment must be for these transgressions. At its starkest the religious life consists of God and the excesses of His creation. And when we judge other people as being excessive we have got this knowledge from Him if we are believers. God, by definition, is not excessive, only we are.

But if we are not believers we are struck by two things: first, that deities seem to be by definition excessive – excessively punitive, excessively loving, excessively demanding and excessively in need of people's devotion; and second, that religious believers, even moderate ones, seem to have excessive confidence in their gods, and are excessively eager to please them, not to mention excuse their apparent failings. The more extreme sceptics of religion, often in patronizing ways, find the whole thing rather childish; as if religious believers – that is, most of the people who have ever lived – are just people who have never got over being frightened of their parents, people who couldn't bear the thought of losing their parents' love and protection. But where do the sceptics get their knowledge of what is excessive from? How does anyone know what too much belief is? Isn't the thing about religious belief that you can't have too much of it? Just as the thing about being sceptical is that you can never be sceptical enough; in deciding what to believe we need to keep our wits about us. Do we believe too much in science now? We call people religious fanatics when they believe things that we don't, and when they believe things in ways that we don't. God is not called a religious fanatic by the people who believe in Him. Islamic fundamentalists think that we believe too much in democratic freedoms and consumer capitalism; we think they believe too much in Islam. It is the hope of modern liberals that we can all talk about the things that matter most to us without losing our tempers or killing people. Do we believe this too much?

What mattered most to most people, until very recently, was their relationship with their gods; and gods, traditionally, have been to die for; one of the things people have been able to do, in the name of religion, is sacrifice their lives and the lives of others. If we think this is excessive – if we are horrified by suicide bombers in the Middle East, or Buddhist monks setting fire to themselves in Vietnam – are we saying anything more than, this is absolutely unacceptable behaviour and we must do what we can to prevent it? In other words, are we using the idea of excess as a kind of rhetorical ploy to say we don't want this to happen, that it makes us feel things we can't bear to feel? What people use their religious beliefs to do – what they do in the name of their religions – might make us wonder not simply, what should we believe, but what kind of thing is a belief? Clearly a belief can be something that permits you to kill people. Our religious beliefs may be the tools we use to manage – to legitimate and contain – the excesses of our nature.

So, from a psychoanalytic point of view, we can't only say, as Freud did, that religion is for people who are frightened of growing up. We must also say that we have delegated to a figure called God all the excesses we find most troubling in ourselves, which broadly speaking are our excessive love for ourselves and others, and our excessive punitiveness. God in this view carries the part of ourselves that asks too much of us, that is endlessly demanding, that wants us to be more or better than we are; that is, in short, excessively moralistic.

But God is also the figure for whom we are not too much. God provides the ultimate reassurance that our lives are not too much for us, not more than we can bear, which is something we are all prone to feel. So without God we can feel uncontained. If God is dead everything is permitted; this is a frightening thought partly because when God was alive everything seems to have been permitted. When Dostoyevsky wrote 'if God doesn't exist, everything is permitted' he implied that without God we will be even more excessive than we have already been. God is there to set limits, so we must experience ourselves as potentially limitless, as too much for ourselves. It is as though we can't bear the complexity of our own minds, with their competing needs and desires and beliefs and feelings. It could be something of a relief to imagine that one could narrow one's mind, be more single-minded, more focused; become, in Wallace Stevens's phrase, 'the emperor of one idea'.

Adam and Eve were interested in two ideas: they were interested in God and obeying His law; and they were interested in the knowledge He had forbidden them (God, of course, may have made them excessively interested in this knowledge by forbidding it). What Milton called 'their excess', for the religious sceptic, was their way to freedom; for the believer it was their way to sin and death. Whether or not we are Christians, the fundamental problem of our own tendencies towards excess began by there being a religious solution. Religions are either what we have invented and recruited to deal with our excess, the excesses of our desire and our vulnerability met by the omniscience and omnipotence of our gods and their laws; or our religions have been more of the problem, rather than the solution. Instead of being tyrannized by our needs and the scarcity of our resources, we are tyrannized by our gods and our laws, and our belief in them; the cured alcoholic becomes addicted to Alcoholics

Anonymous, one excess replacing another. So it is also worth asking what our excesses may be a solution to, or an attempted solution to: what is the problem that our excesses are trying to solve? And this, I think, is where what we call religious fanaticism is particularly instructive.

It is, of course, excessive in the most misleading way to suggest that all religious fanatics are the same, or even similar; even describing someone as a religious fanatic puts one in the position of supposedly knowing what the right way to believe is. A 'fanatic', the Anglican *Oxford English Dictionary* tells us, is someone 'inspired' or 'possessed' by 'a deity or demon', someone 'frenzied', someone 'affected by excessive and mistaken enthusiasm'; clearly not our kind of person. I want to presume that religious fanatics are people who are willing to do whatever harm is necessary to protect and promote their religious beliefs, which are the things that matter most to them in their lives. What might make someone believe and behave in this way (many people, incidentally, feel similarly about their children, but they are not called 'children fanatics')? There are, I think, three possible ways of accounting for what we call religious fanaticism. First, that excessive belief is called up to stifle excessive doubt, as if the fanatic is saying to himself: 'If I don't continually prove my belief in this extreme way, what will be revealed is my extreme faithlessness, or despair, or confusion, or even emptiness.' Supreme conviction is a self-cure for an infestation of doubts. We could call this 'excess as reassurance'; where there are excessive acts there are excessive uncertainties. Or, second, excessive acts of belief are required to persuade other people, as if the fanatic is saying to himself: 'What matters most in the world to me will not be listened to, or considered, or thought about or even noticed unless a dramatic statement is made.' We could call this excess to ensure recognition; wherever there are excessive acts there are excessive fears about invisibility, excessive doubts about people's attention. In both these accounts you will notice that the religious fanatic is described as a kind of strategist, as a person with a project; as someone who knows what they want to say, what they want to achieve. Being excessive in words or actions, in inflammatory rhetoric or violent actions, is a form of communication; conversion by other means What the religious fanatic knows is just how contagious excess can be; excessive words and actions are haunting, they make one's presence felt; they make people excessive in their responses. Priests, Nietzsche writes, 'have shown almost inexhaustible ingenuity in exploring the implications of this one question: how is an excess of emotion to be attained?' If you can make people excessively emotional you can manipulate them; and one of the best ways of making them excessively emotional is to do something excessive to them. Suicide bombers don't convert people but they make the existence of their religion unforgettable, undismissible.

There is, though, a third possibility, the one that I want to end on because it seems to me potentially the most interesting, though perhaps the most daunting; and this is that the religious fanatic is someone for whom something about themselves and their lives is too much; and because not knowing what that is is so disturbing they need to locate it as soon as possible. And this is where culture comes in with its supply of ready-mades. Because the state of frustration cannot be borne – because, perhaps, it is literally unbearable, as long-term personal and political injustice always is – it requires an extreme solution, which is usually a fast one. How someone comes to believe something is more revealing than what they believe. In this account our excessive behaviour shows us how obscure we are to ourselves and how we obscure ourselves; how our frustrations, odd as this may seem, are excessively difficult to locate, to formulate. Wherever and whenever we are excessive in our lives it is the sign of an as yet unknown deprivation. Fanatics are people who have had to wait too long for something that may not exist. Wherever there is an excessive frustration there is a false solution; this would be an excessive way of putting it. Our excesses are the best clues we have to our own poverty; and our best way of concealing it from ourselves.

On What is Fundamental

The fact that there are things we do care
about is plainly more basic to us – more
constitutive of our essential nature – than
what those things are.

Harry G. Frankfurt, *Taking Ourselves
Seriously and Getting It Right*

Whatever is held to be of fundamental importance,
of fundamental value, cannot by definition be treated
casually. Indeed, one of the ways we recognize the
fundamental things when they turn up in conversation is that people tend to lose their composure when
they talk about them. An obvious rule of thumb
would be: people become violent, lose their civility,
when something that is fundamental to them is felt
to be under threat. And what psychoanalysis adds to
this is that fundamental things sometimes get displaced – that when we are talking about pornography, say, we may also be talking about our anxieties
about what was going on inside our mothers' bodies;
we can't be as sure as we would like to be that we

always know what we are arguing about. If we have education, as Robert Frost said, so that we can listen to other people without losing our tempers, then we can't help but notice that education doesn't always work around the fundamental things; no amount of education will stop you getting heated up when you fall in love, or your child gets ill, or you start having a conversation about the State of Israel. The fundamental things are the things that upset us; and even though we think of our civility as constituted by our fundamental beliefs, our civility and our fundamental beliefs are easily at odds with one another. We kill people to defend our virtues, not our vices.

More people than ever before have views now about fundamentalism, and views about the holding of strong beliefs; both what kind of experience belief is, and what believing must or should entail. And one of the things we need to work out now is how we think we know about fundamentalism at all; and how we go about finding out about these things, and how we get to speak about them. And this applies, of course, to people brought up within the traditional faiths, and those who have drifted away from them. In everyone's history there are likely to have been people who were strong believers; people who could not have conceived of themselves – who could not have conceived of anything – without their relationship to their God or gods.

Because we tend to think of fundamentalism in

the light of recent events we are more likely than ever before to be thinking of Muslim fundamentalism. And for those of us who are not Muslims, and for some of us who are, this means realizing how little we know; and that if we want to know anything we are going to have to read books and talk to people about our ignorance. For most white non-Muslim westerners knowledge of Islam, let alone knowledge of Islamic fundamentalism, is going to be at once academic and sensationalist, derived from reading books by so-called experts, watching the news and reading reports by journalists. Of course, Christian fundamentalism, defined by the *Oxford English Dictionary* as 'strict adherence to traditional orthodox tenets (e.g., the literal inerrancy of Scripture) held to be fundamental to the Christian faith: opposed to liberalism and modernism', is something known, or rather known about, by many of us. But at least for many of us, Christian fundamentalism is something about which we have usually pejorative and caricatural associations, and is not something we have lived; we can become informed about these increasingly prominent fundamentalisms, but we haven't lived them yet.

And yet, of course – and this is the kind of move that psychoanalysis has made all too available to us – we are all fundamentalists about something. There must be, psychoanalysis might tell us, to put it in as silly a way as possible, a fundamentalist in all of us;

we may think of ourselves consciously so to speak as liberals and modernists, but what these relatively new forms of self-description are up against is a more old-fashioned, even archaic inner fundamentalist. The psychoanalytical way of talking would make this inner fundamentalism something that we liberals and modernists should ideally have outgrown. There is, we should note, always a progress myth around when we liberals and modernists – and the psychoanalytically minded – talk about fundamentalists. Fundamentalists, even though none of us would wish perhaps to put it this way, will seem to many of us to be suffering from a regressive fixation. They are, as homosexuals were once supposed to be, deprived of something: affluence, liberal education, democracy, good-enough mothering, strong fathers, and so on. Fundamentalism is not one of our ego-ideals; we don't want our children to become fundamentalists, and we can give good reasons for this derived from our liberal quasi-modernist traditions. Extremism, except when it is artistic vocationism and parental passion, is something that we have learned to be extremely wary of. You can be fanatical about your children's well-being, indeed you should be; and you can be inflexible in your need to paint, say, or to write. But insofar as we can divide up the realms, you must not be what we would call a fanatic in your erotic life, or in your political or religious views. Once you become a fanatic – someone who, literally or metaphorically, believes in the literal inerrancy of your scripture (or your so-called sexual perversion), you change from being (in the language of the political philosopher Chantal Mouffe) an adversary into being an enemy and thus cease to be someone with whom one can have the kind of productive conflict that Mouffe believes democracy depends upon.

And, indeed, when we think of fundamentalism now we think of it, as we have been encouraged to think of it, as the enemy of democracy. For the fundamentalist, to debate is to miss the point. In the conciliation of rival claims, our preferred form of political life, there are rival claims that the fundamentalist cannot consider. But the democrat, like the fundamentalist, also always has to decide which are the inadmissible claims. We democrats believe that the fundamentalist claim is inadmissible. And yet it would be misleading to say that the democrat believes that everything is negotiable, that all views should be considered. All contemporary liberal democracies set limits to free speech around incitement to racial hatred and incitement to harm. There is, to use the title of Stanley Fish's salutary book, *No Such Thing as Free Speech: And It's a Good Thing Too*; in Fish's words, 'the line between what is permitted and what is spurned is always being drawn and redrawn, and structures of constraint are simultaneously always in place and always subject to revision

if the times call for it and resources are up to it'. For
the fundamentalist, who in Fish's terms is different
in degree but not in kind from the democrat, the
line between what is permitted and what is spurned
has either been drawn once and for all, or can only
ever be redrawn to a small degree, by a small number
of 'legitimate' people. For the fundamentalist, at
least in our cartoon version of him – and he is usually but not always a he – the structures of constraint
are by definition not always being drawn and
redrawn, are not subject to whim or circumstance or
competing vested interests. For the fundamentalist,
in this sense, there can be no such thing as progress,
except perhaps the progress of keeping things as
they are, under pressure: under the pressure of secu-
larization, globalization, modernization. 'There is
no such thing as free speech,' Fish writes, 'because
from the very start your sense of just how free speech
should be is shadowed by your identification of, and
obligation to, the good in whose name acts of speech
are to be justified.' We are free to speak so long as
what we say serves, rather than sabotages, our core
values. Whatever is being said, someone is always
being reassured about something. For the fundamentalist, as for the democrat, people can say what
they like; but when they start saying things that aim
to destroy the foundational preconditions of their
given political culture there have to be penalties.
After all, what would it mean to value something,

and not want to protect it? If democrats really value dissent, competing claims, rival views, what would it say about the nature of their commitment, the nature of their belief, if they allowed these things to be violated? And the same, of course, holds for the fundamentalist. It becomes a question of what valuing people, or ideals, involves, and might involve us in. It's not incidental that belief is usually linked with violence. People are prepared to die and kill for other people, and for other people's sentences. So the other question is something like: what is our picture of a core belief, or an absolute value? How do we imagine that these things work inside us and between us such that we are willing to make the ultimate sacrifice of our lives for them? If there are beliefs, or descriptions, that are fundamental to our sense of who we are, and the kind of lives we want, why would we do anything other than everything to protect them? What kinds of things are beliefs if we are willing to exchange them for other beliefs?

If something is fundamental we should assume that it is not subject to redescription. If we take our initial, cursory definition of fundamentalism from the nineteenth-century Anglican *Oxford English Dictionary* as 'the literal inerrancy of Scripture' we might take this to be saying that there are people who think of themselves as conveying or transmitting the truth of their scripture, but that for these people the truth of their scripture is beyond dispute. To dispute it would be to misunderstand it; to think of it as open to interpretation except by the qualified few would be to treat it as something that it is not. It would be a category error. If I read the New Testament as a fiction akin to other fictions – as a kind of novel or series of short stories – then from the fundamentalist point of view this is not what I might want to call a misrecognition but a sin. The Christian might say, the charitable Christian, that I am resisting the message of the gospel; that I am in no state to receive the good news. Because the fundamentalist knows the truth of his revelation, its inerrancy, he knows by the same token the status of those who do not share his belief. The issues here are so grave that no one is going to 'agree to differ'. The best that can be hoped for, from the liberalism side – and even this sounds optimistic in our present predicament – is what the political philosopher John Gray calls modus vivendi. 'We can think of the liberal project,' he writes in *Two Faces of Liberalism*:

> not as aiming to found a universal regime or way of life but as the pursuit of modus vivendi among different regimes and ways of life. If we think of it in this way, liberalism is not a partisan claim for the universal authority of a particular morality, but the search for terms of coexistence between different moralities. In this alternative view, liberalism has to do with handling the conflicts of cultures that will always be different, not founding a universal civilization.

The project, Gray writes, is coexistence not consensus, even if coexistence has already begun to sound like just one more Utopian ideal. But clearly, from a psychoanalytic or Freudian perspective, Gray's description sounds germane. In Freud's account of the divided modern subject there can be no consensus between the conflicting agencies, no universal regime or way of life shared by the so-called id, ego and super-ego. It is indeed the search for terms of coexistence between different moralities that is as good a description as any of the psychoanalytic project, what Lacan calls 'the psychoanalytic opportunity'. What is fundamental in the Freudian picture of the psyche is the inevitability, and therefore the necessity, of conflict. And what is also fundamental – and linked to this – is the idea of resistance. In every psychoanalysis the patient and the analyst come up against something in the patient – and something in the analyst – that is un-negotiable. Whatever is un-negotiable in the patient, wherever nothing can be exchanged, wherever the greatest violence is unleashed in the patient, that is where what we might call the patient's fundamentalism is. And it can also be, by the same token, where the analysis begins, what the analysis is about: or, indeed, where it stalls. The conundrum here, though, is which, in these terms, is the fundamentalist, the one who can recognize a resistance or the one who resists? We can, of course, recognize the signs of a resistance without

knowing what it is that is being resisted. Those who
already know what is being resisted – who already
know what there is to resist – may be akin to fundamentalists (psychoanalysts are, after all, people who
have to be more interested in psychoanalysis than in
other people). But so is the patient at the point at
which he will have none of what the analyst is saying. In psychoanalysis, as in all so-called relationships, we always find a clash of fundamentalisms,
conflicts about what is fundamental, and what it is to
acknowledge these fundamentals. In this sense,
people always meet each other, people come across
each other, at an impasse. And this in itself may make
the psychoanalytic situation a useful site for the consideration of what we may be talking about – at an
ordinary, even at a secular, level – when we talk, in
our mostly unknowing way, about fundamentalism.
We may not need to find out about it, to inform
ourselves as we should, because we already know
too much about it; even if we are not what John
Gray calls enlightenment fundamentalists. (It is not
incidental, of course, that fundamentalists fascinate
us: we are never indifferent to them.) It may be
worth, I think, going back to the old-fashioned and
unfashionable topic of defences, and of defences as
forms of acknowledgement. It is not incidental, as
many people have pointed out, that the history of
psychoanalysis is also the history of the rise of fascism
and nationalism in Western Europe. Whatever else

Freud's work is, it is an attempt to describe what the modern individual is up against in himself and with others; it is about the self-protective modern individual. The individual who doesn't (and does) want to get too close to the things and people that excite him. And psychoanalysis itself, it should be noted, is something people have always got very excited about, and have always prided themselves on dismissing.

One thing that the modernist liberal and the fundamentalist may be said to share is what psychoanalysts after Freud call a resistance: each believes that there is something the other refuses to see that is considered to be true, or at least better. Were the other side capable of the requisite acknowledgement, both of them believe, the world would be as it should be. We would be living the lives we are required to live – required, that is, by God, or the relevant set of secular beliefs and authorities. It is, though, a situation in which persuasion, negotiation and even discussion keep breaking down; here, we modern liberals might say, words no longer work in the way we want them to; here we come up against the real difficulty of changing people. It is, of course, a version of the feeling that most couples have at one time or another, that there is, as we say, no point in talking. It is like what happens when the teacher is unable to teach the child. The question then becomes, at least for people like us: what can we usefully say about that situation in

which there is no point in talking? The talking cure
turned up to show us what talking cannot cure. We
might believe in what we call discussion and debate,
progress and difference, and so on; but others might
believe in revelation and tradition, in authority and
purity, and so on. We are talking about the moment
in which people begin to believe, in despair or with
relief, that coexistence rather than consensus is our
best option; or alternatively believe that the unbelievers – those who are not of the same mind – must
be eradicated. Coexistence, in other words, is the
modern liberal's last hope; the only remaining political ideal left, and one that will survive only if that
is itself agreed upon. Those who do not believe in
coexistence – those who value their fundamental
beliefs over their own lives – will not want to try
to work out what the preconditions might be for
coexistence.

There is clearly a risk in negotiating with those for
whom negotiation is itself sinful, with those who
don't think that we live by trading with the enemy
but that we live by exterminating the enemy. When
we negotiate with such people we – wittingly or
unwittingly – collude with our own destruction.
'Religious moderates,' Sam Harris writes in *The End
of Faith*,

> are, in large part, responsible for the religious con-
> flicts in our world, because their beliefs provide the

context in which scriptural literalism and religious violence can never be adequately opposed.

This acknowledges the problem, but runs the risk of protracting it; religious moderates, by being moderate, appease religious fanatics and by so doing allow them to flourish. And yet Harris can't, by definition, be proposing that we meet fire with fire, religious violence with religious violence. The perennial post-enlightenment question is: what is it to adequately oppose scriptural literalism and the religious violence it often entails? Can we avoid violating our core beliefs in the ways we defend them? When we bully the bullies we are, in both senses, betraying ourselves. If it is integral to someone's belief that they should destroy you, what do you say to them; or, rather more realistically, what do you do with them? You can imitate your enemy by trying to destroy him; or you can settle into a permanent project of doing what you can both to limit his power over you and to protect yourself from him.

It will be obvious to anyone who is psychoanalytically minded that Freud's so-called model of the mind is a cartoon of precisely this predicament: the ego of Freud's modern individual is pitted against two fanatics, the super-ego and the id, both agencies without scepticism about their own commitments; both fundamentalists in the definition of Lord May, the zoologist and ex-president of the Royal Society. Fundamentalism, he said, doesn't necessarily derive from sacred texts. It's where a belief trumps a fact and refuses to confront the facts. All ideas should be open to questioning, and the merit of ideas should be assessed on the strength of evidence that supports them and not on the credentials or affiliations of the individuals proposing them. It is not a recipe for the comfortable life, but it is demonstrably a powerful engine for understanding how the world actually works and for applying this understanding.

(Lord May's outgoing speech to the Royal Society,
reported in the *Guardian,* 30 November 2005)

Science, we have been told for some time, is the best antidote to fundamentalism; and yet science has to believe that it can only ever fail by its own criteria. But in the Freudian schema, one might say, the id has desires that trump the facts and the super-ego – the 'obscene' super-ego as Lacan calls it – has beliefs that do so. The 'drives' of the id are, in this picture, the fundamental promptings of our being, the super-ego the fundamental promptings of our being in culture. In psychoanalytic treatment the ideas, the representations of the id and the super-ego, are, in Lord May's words, open to questioning and are, in a sense, assessed on the strength of evidence that supports them. (Evidence can't speak for itself.) But it is what Freud calls the ego that has the task of creating the context in which moral literalism and instinctual violence can be adequately opposed (to rephrase Sam Harris's words). What Freud calls the ego, I want to suggest, is an experiment in imagining, in describing what in ourselves may be available to manage the prevailing forms of fundamentalism in which we live and have our being. After all, what we now call fundamentalism was until very recently a version of what people were likely to call religious belief.

If one way of describing Freud's so-called model of the mind is as a war of contending fundamentalisms — the non-scriptural biologically based drives of the id, and the scriptural, if only partly read, moral dictates of the super-ego — then we may usefully be able to see the ego as Freud's device for thinking about ways of bearing the fundamentalisms that are the inheritance of the modern Western individual. The ego, one might say, is a modernist fictional character trying to live as well, as satisfyingly, as he can, informed by potentially murderous convictions and desires. And the astounding thing is that Freud believes that there is this part, this version of the self that does manage things. Freud may have famously said, vis-à-vis the ego, that the rider has to guide the horse in the direction that the horse wants to go in: that the ego is not master in his own house, and so on; and yet he also believed, albeit ambivalently, that there was a social practice called psychoanalysis that could help the so-called patient, and this was by the analyst forming what he called an alliance with the

patient's ego. There were the intractable determin-
isms of the drives and traditional inherited morality
and there was, or there might be, this something else,
the ego, that has of course been the object of so much
suspicion. It has been, perhaps unsurprisingly, the
ego that psychoanalysts after Freud have argued over,
its provenance, its function and its power. Freud, in
other words, is wondering, through the fictions of
psychoanalysis, whether there is anything more to
the modern individual, anything other than this war
of fundamentals that always pre-exist the individual
and into which he was born. Freud wants to know
what extremes modern people are subject to, and
why we don't want to describe ourselves as extrem-
ists. Freud's work is part of the post-enlightenment
project of working out what we can be if we are not
fanatics, or whether this in itself is the ultimate illusion of the progressivist modern individual. It might
be part of this project, which I think psychoanalysis
is party to, to give an account of a good life that
would not entail beliefs to kill, die or torture for.
When Freud in his late work *Civilization and Its Dis-
contents* referred to Eros as having the 'task ... of
uniting separate individuals into a community bound
together by libidinal ties' he was alluding to this as
one half of his equation of what he took to be the
human essence, the war between Thanatos and Eros.

But as I say, it is the ego in the Freudian topog-
raphy that is delegated this unpromising task of

making the fundamentalisms survivable. And it is of obvious and pertinent historical interest that the early *fin de siècle* Freud – the Freud of the great early works: *Studies in Hysteria, Three Essays on Sexuality, The Joke Book, The Dream Book* and *The Psychopathology of Everyday Life* – is more of an id-psychologist, keener to tell us stories about the vicissitudes of sexual desire; whereas the later Freud, the Freud of the First World War and its aftermath, is more of an ego-psychologist, keener to tell us stories about the ego's resources in the face of what Laplanche was to call 'the attack of the drives on the ego', and especially the aggressive drives; and about why psychoanalysis was so difficult. And within fifteen years of the end of the Second World War there was the attack of the critics on the ego, in which the fundamental question was asked as to whether a strong ego was the problem or the solution in the suffering of the modern individual. Was psychoanalysis an enlightenment humanism, or an anti-humanism? Was the project to be as kind as possible, as Kleinians would suggest, or as truly desirous as possible, as the Lacanians would preach? Was the well-analysed analyst, as Lacan said, more likely to fall in love with his patient, or less likely, as every other school of analysis would assert? The question in psychoanalysis, as in the wider culture, became: who, if anyone, is in charge in the modern individual? Is our essence such that the notion of self-control, or indeed the notion of a self,

or a will, are any longer plausible? Is it, indeed, the
very nature of the so-called ego to be plausible – to
itself and others – and is this the fundamental
self-deception? What, after all, are we going to
replace plausibility with? And is it indeed not the
function of the essence – a description of what is
fundamental to your being – to give us plausibility?
To put it as schematically as possible, the Freudian
ego was either, in Lacan's terms, an alienated structure, the site of the subject's misrecognition of itself,
or it was, in the various ego-psychologies, the individual's only hope for a viable life. The ego is by
definition embattled, but it is only the ego that is
capable of keeping the show on the road. 'The Ego
is victorious,' Anna Freud writes in the conclusion
to her great book *The Ego and the Mechanisms of
Defence*,

> when its defensive measures effect their purpose,
> i.e., when they enable it to restrict the development
> of anxiety and unpleasure and so to transform the
> instincts that, even in difficult circumstances, some
> measure of gratification is secured, thereby establish-
> ing the most harmonious relations possible between
> the id, the super-ego and the forces of the outside
> world.

Written in 1936, this sounds now like a kind of stoical
optimism; the modern individual's aim is, in her

measured phrase, 'some measure of gratification', and this is achieved by the ego's restricting, not controlling, the id, the super-ego and the forces of the outside world. These, from a classical psychoanalytic point of view, are the three fundamentals. It is implied, though, puzzling as this may seem, that the ego has some agency, some freedom, some choice, all the things the post-enlightenment person thinks of as essential to his being. The intractable, the unnegotiable, is everywhere and yet there is, wished for or not, a margin of opportunity; and it is here that gratification is secured. The ego has what Anna Freud calls 'the faculty of self-observation'; the creature that can reflect on itself, it is hoped, is the creature who can thereby transform itself. And it is hoped, by the same token, that the creature that can reflect on itself will be inclined to temper its desire. The id and the super-ego can be observed but are not themselves observers. They are blind in the sense that they are not seeking to in any way transform themselves; they are akin to fundamentalists in that they are not seeking to change, contest or doubt their own projects (the super-ego – our internal voice of self-reproach – has a notably limited and repetitive vocabulary). Rather like us secular, liberal moderns observing in some trepidation the fundamentalisms of the East and the West, the ego sees itself as the one who establishes – who looks for – the most harmonious relations possible; like the ego we see ourselves as the only ones capable of observation and reflection while they blindly go their violent, self-righteous ways. A democrat in a world of fascists, the ego wants, indeed needs, everyone to have a voice without anyone taking over; a 'victory' for the ego is not the defeat of the id or the super-ego but merely their restriction. It is supposedly a civilizing process – where id was there ego shall be – and the uncivilized are those who are not seeking exchange, those not interested in establishing the most harmonious relations possible. In this context the ego, one could say, is Freud's most radical creation, his most modern, progressivist fiction; the id and the super-ego – and in a different sense, the external world – are versions of old-fashioned fundamentalists, voices telling you the absolute truth about yourself, what you need, what you believe, what you are, what you can and can't do. They are voices of 'literal inerrancy'; then something new, modern, turns up saying that we can reflect on these voices, that there are voices that can compete with these fundamentalist voices, that it is possible to live a non-servile life, a life without domination, a life without 'strict adherence to traditional orthodox tenets'. That, in short, where fundamentalism was, there rationality can be; where revelation and scripture was, there conversation can be. Psychoanalysis, as a product of its times, asks a simple question: are there voices in the modern individual that are not fundamentalist, and what do they sound like?

And this, it is important to notice, is different from the question of whether there are voices that are anti-fundamentalist. There are the voices we have to deal with the fundamentalists in ourselves; and there are the voices that are not fundamentalist. This may be a distinction that psychoanalysis, as a listening cure, can help us with.

The Freudian ego, the ego as described by Freud and his daughter, is so busy, like ourselves contending with the fundamentalists — protecting its pleasure and ideals through sufficient defensiveness — that it has little time for the non-fundamentalist voice. Indeed, one way of formulating the conflict about ego-psychology that is symptomatic of a wider cultural unease would be to wonder whether it is possible for the ego not to become a fundamentalist itself in its battle with the fundamentalisms; is it possible, in other words, for the ego so described not to be the fundamentalist of its own preferred image of itself, not to be fanatical about the recognitions it requires?

In a recent summary in his book *Sex on the Couch* the philosopher Richard Boothby gives a useful account of the way the Freudian ego works at its definition. 'The ego functions,' he writes,

> to categorize things and persons in the outside world
> (those with whom I identify versus those with whom
> I conflict), but even more importantly the ego

discriminates between contending forces of my own
desire (those of my impulses on which I will act ver-
sus those which I will refuse and repress). Fundamental to this conception of psychic structure is Freud's
assumption that we are animated by a great heteroge-
neity of impulses. We are, at some basic level of ourselves, a chaos of conflicting urges. Ego thus refers to
the restricted economy of impulses that grounds my
feeling of having a stable and predictable identity.
The ego selects from a range of impulse energies and
leaves the others behind. 'Id' names the remainder of
my urges and incipient acts that have been excluded
from the ego and held in repression.

Boothby, like Anna Freud, refers to the ego as
restricting – 'ego thus refers to the restricted economy of impulses' – not dominating or controlling;
the ego here categorizes, discriminates and selects,
all in the service of sustaining a 'feeling of having a
stable and predictable identity'. The ego simplifies
the self in the service of survival. But in order to do
this, of course, it must know beforehand, as it were,
which impulses are the unnecessarily disruptive ones.
In other words the ego is presented here, as often in
Freud, as in some way mysteriously knowing about
its own nature; it can spot an impulse that will ruin
my feeling of having a stable and predictable identity, and will have the power, to some extent, to
repress it. Like a peculiarly refined aesthete the ego is

here selecting the impulses that will make him who
he wants to be. How, one might ask, is this different
from the fundamentalisms we have been describing?
The fundamentalist must be by definition the person
who knows exactly what he wants (even if this
is described in terms of what God wants for him).
The phrase 'a stable and predictable identity', like the
phrase 'the most harmonious relations possible', is
not incompatible with the notion of 'strict adherence
to traditional orthodox tenets'. It is as though the ego
must already know what it must adhere to – even
though it is not strictly speaking a tenet – to sustain
itself. That, one could say, is what is fundamental;
the belief that I always already know what I want. In
psychoanalytic language this is the belief of someone in a perverse state of mind. What I am calling the
non-fundamentalist voice does not know beforehand
what it wants; does not think of itself as equipped
with any kind of text, or anything akin to a text, that
can give it such knowledge, such guidance, such orientation. If to believe in something (or someone) is to
know what you want, and what we call fundamentalism is an extreme version of this knowing – so
extreme indeed that people will kill and die for it –
then in talking about alternatives to fundamentalism
we are talking about finding different forms of wanting. It is what we might call their forms of wanting
that people are not keen to give up. What is fundamental, in psychoanalytic language, is the ways in

which we do our wanting. And it is this that the Freudian ego is supposed to fashion.

It would be misleading to suggest, or even to imply, that the language of psychoanalysis provides some kind of answer to what we liberals think of as the problem of fundamentalism, and fundamentalists think of as the problem we liberals have. You will have noticed that at times I have used the words 'fundamentalist', 'fanatic' and 'extremist' as though they were interchangeable – as, indeed, the popular and tabloid press use them – which they are not; and I have used the word 'we' to refer to all those people who are opposed, as though there was a consensus among them, which there is not. Indeed, the only thing the available generalizations about fundamentalism share – and the word seems to have been first used in the early twentieth century by Protestants in Southern California – is the sense that the various fundamentalisms have been reactions to, and not simply refusals of, modernization. As, of course, was psychoanalysis, which needs to be seen as another site – another language – in which these issues are considered (and which is potentially itself another fundamentalism). Fundamentalism, in the sense in which contemporaries use the word, is, in Karen Armstrong's good popularizing words from *The Battle for God*,

> a reaction against the scientific and secular culture that first appeared in the West, but which has since

taken root in other parts of the world. The West has developed an entirely unprecedented and wholly different type of civilization, so the religious response to it has been unique. The fundamentalist movements that have evolved in our own day have a symbiotic relationship with modernity. They may reject the scientific rationalism of the West but they cannot escape it. Western civilization has changed the world. Nothing – including religion – can ever be the same again. All over the globe people have been struggling with these new conditions and have been forced to reassess their religious traditions, which were designed for an entirely different type of society.

Freud, at his most explicit, was part of the enlightenment attempt to debunk religion through disproof. But perhaps more interestingly, he displaced the problem that Armstrong and many other commentators refer to as at the heart of modernity, the dismantling of traditional societies. Where Armstrong refers to people having to struggle with new conditions of secular rationalism and global markets, 'forced to reassess their religious traditions, which were designed for an entirely different type of society', Freud talks of people being forced to reassess their childhoods, which were designed for an entirely different type of society. In other words, for religious tradition Freud reads infantile sexuality with the Oedipus complex at its heart, with Freud describing the modern individual resisting at all costs the modernity of adulthood. And the Freudian patient, above all, has to make conscious, has to articulate, the earlier ways of wanting that have organized his life. Growing up, in Freud's description, is a parable of this transition modern individuals have had to make from religious traditionalism to secular modernity, in which something akin to fundamentalist desire for and adoration of the parents and the family have to be replaced by something else and hopefully in the process made less frantic. In the Freudian story the developing individual has to sacrifice her heart's desire (for the parents) for a poor but supposedly more promising substitute.

Psychoanalysis, in short, is another language to redescribe what we think of as fundamental, and the fundamentalism that attends such urgencies. The way in which we can see psychoanalysis as another place in which these pressing issues are played out is further illuminated by Malise Ruthven's account of what he calls a 'benchmark' in the development of modern fundamentalisms. There is, he writes in *Fundamentalism: The Search for Meaning*, a

> transition from traditionalism to fundamentalism, the point where traditionalism becomes self-consciously reactive. Whereas the true traditionalist does not know he is a traditionalist, the fundamentalist is forced by

the logic of his desire to defend tradition into making strategic selections. Textual anomalies are either denied, or subsumed into the hermeneutics of inerrancy, where the burden of proof is shifted from God to humanity. They can then be explained as errors of human understanding, rather than flaws in the text itself.

Just as the true traditionalist doesn't know he is a traditionalist, in the Freudian account the child does not know that he is a child; and then something happens – call it growing up or the Oedipus complex, or the birth of a sibling – and he becomes self-consciously reactive. He will defend to the death, usually through symptoms, his childhood wishes. The fundamentalist is forced, as Ruthven writes, by the logic of his desire to defend tradition; the Freudian adult is forced by the logic of his desire to defend his childhood ethos. When new wants, when new forms of wanting, are imposed upon the modern individual, there is often violent resistance, a more militant recreation of the past. At its starkest it is a simple picture: something from the past, without which life is not bearable, runs the risk of being both destroyed and replaced. Both sides in this mortal conflict believe that they are the guardians (and prophets) of the only viable future. It would be literally nonsensical or evil to compromise on these issues. Our relationship to a selected past is each group's defining characteristic; without it their group no longer exists.

When we talk about these issues in this way our liberal vocabulary begins to sound meagre; words like 'compromise', 'negotiation', 'discussion', 'persuasion', 'progress' – unmoored from any shared ground for disagreement – seem feeble. What kind of compromise would we hope to reach with a convicted racist? How might we persuade a Palestinian that the Israelis are well-meaning? What would we discuss with a suicide bomber? What would be progress, from both points of view, in discussing the meaning of life with a born-again Christian? It is as though the project of civil influence, of coexistence, of the conciliating of rival claims, is plausible only if you keep the hard cases out of the picture. 'Dialogue' between, say, the capitalist fundamentalism of the West and Islamic fundamentalism sounds like the kind of thing that could only be dreamed up by people working in universities, or people who watch the news and hope for the best. It is as though we have had the wrong picture of what people are really like; of what people are really like about those things that they take to be fundamental. Having seen the strife between people, the unfathomable conflict they can elicit in each other, we have replaced this perception with fantasies of harmony. The more horrified we are, the more committed we become to the dream of unity. People can get on with each other, but not for very long; and more and more we see that people can't bear each other. We don't want to kill the person we hate most, the psychoanalyst Ernest Jones once remarked, we want to kill the person who arouses in us the most unbearable conflict. More and more people now are living lives of unbearable conflict.

What fundamentalism highlights for us – if only as a phrase – is the question of what is fundamental for us, and what a good relation would be to these fundamental things; what kind of connection we have to the things that matter most to us, both consciously and unconsciously. Freud's contribution to this modern conversation was to say that, in the first instance, what is fundamental to us is our survival, both physical and psychical; and after that, the fundamental thing is instinctual gratification under the aegis of the Oedipus complex. But he also showed us – and this, in its way, is more useful – that we are most resistant to talking about the things that matter most to us. And there is an irony – a reversal of common sense – in this that is worth attending to. We might think: we know what is fundamental, what matters most to us; the only question being whether we can honour these things by abiding by them, by defending them. What Freud suggests, with the language of psychoanalysis, is that we are least willing to apprehend, to acknowledge, to articulate the things that are fundamental to us. There is inerrant scripture, in Freud's view, because we are forever erring around and about our paramount preoccupations. The problem then is, of course, that Freud goes on to tell us what our real, true, deep preoccupations are and so potentially inscribes another scripture where there needn't be one. We are the animals that will kill and be killed for our fundamental beliefs – for the sentences that matter most to us; Freud adds to this that we are the animals committed to never really knowing what our fundamental beliefs are; that where there is conviction there is often the least adequate object. There is something uncanny about how confounding this is; about the effect these ideas can have when they are thought through. The fundamentalist knows who he is; when we speak with our greatest passion about the things that matter most to us it is as if, at least in these moments, we know who we are, or we are something that matters, at least to ourselves; when we are at our most plausible, persuasive, convincing and convinced, Freud adds, we may be at our most defensive. Freud wants us to believe that there is no refuge from our ambivalence, that we identify most with those whom we demonize, but these will be the identifications that we need to keep ourselves unconscious of.

There are versions of the modern self, of the selves we encounter, for whom to discuss, to negotiate, to talk at all is the problem, not the solution; for whom to speak is always to say too much, to endanger the hard-earned familiarity we seem to have with ourselves. It is as if we are also the animals for whom some things — and they are surprisingly often the fundamental things — either cannot or must not be discussed. For whom either there is quite literally an incapacity — some things are just inarticulate; or for whom to speak of such things — to speak of the things that matter most — would entail such potential suffering, such potential loss, that they are to all intents and purposes unspeakable. And psychoanalysis, at its most minimal, tries to clarify this distinction for any given individual (and at its best it tries not to violate the individual's privacy). But we should not be assuming that what is most fundamental to us — whether we are aware of it or not — is necessarily conducive to harmony with ourselves or others. Indeed, we may have to acknowledge, absurd as this might seem, that what is fundamental to us — or the defence of what is fundamental to us — can be the very thing that destroys us. That only what makes our lives worth living is worth dying for. We may of course wonder why values are to die for: why we would want values that make these kinds of demands on us.

There are now a lot of upbeat democratic and rather more low-key psychoanalytic accounts of why conflict is to be valued — as stimulating, as generative, as productive, as truthful, as inclusive, and so on. And fundamentalisms of whatever persuasion at best pay lip-service to the value of conflict and at worst want to abolish it. The fundamentalist of Western capitalism, just like the more ostensibly religious fundamentalists that we hear more about, really believe that the only good life is one in which the enemy, the dissenters, the unpersuaded, are no longer part of the conversation; a world without communists, a world without Jews, a world without unbelievers, is the world as it should be. Those of us who are not drawn to what is loosely, and not so loosely, called fundamentalism; those of us who don't want to be fundamentalist in a war against the fundamentalisms, have a very serious problem. What is the point, after all, of having respect for people who do not respect our respect for them? I don't know what an answer to that question would be; but we are endangered by our optimism.

Sleeping It Off

... our thoughts become true in proportion as they successfully exert their go-between function.

William James, *What Pragmatism Means*

When Bottom says to Titania in *A Midsummer Night's Dream*, 'But, I pray you, let none of your people stir me;/ I have an exposition of sleep come upon me,' we know he is feeling rather tired, and we guess, as the Arden editor helpfully explains, that 'exposition', which is at once an exposing, an expounding and an explaining, is 'a malapropism for "disposition"', which is at once a natural tendency, and a plan for disposing of one's property. The natural inclination to sleep is more likely to come upon one than an explanation of sleep, because sleeping is something we do when we are not aware that that is what we are doing. When we sleep, when we act in plays, when we are under magic spells, we cannot at the same time give an account of what we are doing, without waking up, without breaking the spell. As the play is at pains to show us, we can only be in one place at a time, and yet we are often in two places at once. But what does my waking self have to say about my sleeping self? Not much. We sleep things off but not on, out but not in, as though we think of sleep as a good riddance; as though it helps us to get away from things, rather than to rework them.

It must be from sleep that we get our sense of being here and not being here, of losing ourselves and finding ourselves, of absence and return; and, perhaps most interestingly of all, sleep must be our original and easily lost experience of an absence that is not a form of waiting. Sometimes – though more often as children – we can't wait to wake up, but once we are asleep we are not waiting for anything. Waking up every morning for years on end may reassure us that the lost can be found, that something comes from nothing, that long swathes of experience cannot be remembered because they were never forgotten, that we need to be interrupted, and so on. And yet sleep, unlike what Seamus Heaney calls the 'pre-reflective lived experience' of childhood, is not something we grow out of. It is as though we need to be regularly absent from ourselves, and in a way that cannot be spoken of; we can speak about sleep as a phenomenon – scientists, and the people who see us sleeping, can tell us about how we looked, what we said – but we can never report back about what we did, about what happened, except in the most banal way ('I slept really well', 'I had a bad night', and so on). Sleep, in other words, is a need that we can only experience in, and as, anticipation.

We can experience wanting it, but not having it, the expectation and the aftermath, but never the thing itself. No one will ever say, except in their sleep, 'I'm having a wonderful sleep.' We can sometimes tell the story of our dream but not of the sleep in which we had it; we don't experience dreams as happening in our sleep (nothing about the dream tells us we are sleeping). One of our most intimate and essential activities, sleep can be known about only from someone else. So if we think of sleep as an experience it must radically change our sense of what an experience can be; if we think of it as an object of knowledge, it confirms our dependence on others for such knowledge as is available; and if we think of sleep as an object of desire – and as one of our original paradigms or blueprints for desiring – we may end up radically redescribing the obscurity of such objects. Sleep, after all, is by far the most time-consuming of our earliest desires; and, of course, the only one of those desires that cannot be satisfied by another person (the parent can create the conditions for sleep, but cannot give the child something called sleep). There are two questions: what kind of object of desire is sleep? And what can it tell us about desiring? It would not be strange if sleep was the model for many things that we do. And it would not be strange if we tended not to notice this. Because sleeping is something that we do without knowing that we are doing it.

If sleep is a peculiarly obscure 'obscure object of desire' that is because it is not an object and cannot be located in the external world. If it is anywhere it is inside us as a disposition, as a need, as a process; but unlike other appetites we have to be unconscious for it to be gratified. And we are likely to think of it as a means to an end, not an end in itself; we want what it can give us, but we don't think of it as an exchange, and in this sense our capacity to sleep is a model for our capacity for self-reliance, sleep being the necessary thing we provide for ourselves. Wanting to sleep is wanting something that no one can give you, but that anyone can stop you having.

So as an object of desire sleep is something I always possess, but that I can be prevented by myself and other people from getting to. Other people, including myself, have to collaborate with me to let me not get it, but to let it, in Bottom's words, 'come upon me', come over me. It is not something we can grasp, but something we can only receive. So when people talk about 'grabbing some sleep' they are making a category error: sleep is not a person you can grab. If we took sleep as our preferred picture of an object of desire, began to see desiring as more like desiring sleep, we would be doing things very differently. We would, for example, see satisfaction as something we had to relinquish ourselves for, and we would relish anticipation and longing. And we would never think that reporting back was possible or the point.

Children Behaving Badly

Possibilities are everywhere, only
Access to them barred ...

Stephen Romer, 'Departures'

I Should School Make You Happy?

There is a famous sentence from Thomas Jefferson's
Declaration of Independence that formulates something essential about what most modern liberals
believe about both government and education: 'We
hold these truths to be self-evident & undeniable; that
all men are created equal, that they are endowed
by their Creator with certain unalienable rights, that
among these are Life, Liberty, and the pursuit of happiness.' Some of us might not believe in the Creator part,
and all of us would assume now that by 'men' he means
men and women; and probably none of us would
quibble, though these are very modern, that is, recent,
ideas: that people are born, if not created, equal, and
that they have a right to life and liberty. But what
does it mean to have an unalienable right to the pursuit

of happiness? It is, perhaps we should note, the only thing on his list that is a pursuit. At first sight, it seems to be a pretty good idea; and no one, presumably, would promote the pursuit of unhappiness. If we are convinced of anything these days we are convinced that we are pleasure-seeking creatures, who want to minimize the pain and frustrations of our lives. We are the creatures who, perhaps unlike all other animals, pursue happiness.

But fortunately, and unfortunately, the other thing we know is that pleasure, like happiness, is not as simple a thing as we would like it to be: people can be frightened of pleasure; they can hide from themselves what their real pleasures are; they can use pleasure as a way of avoiding necessary pain (drinking alcohol or taking drugs, for example, to avoid intimacy or the useful and necessary awkwardnesses and difficulties of social life); they can get pleasure from pain – from their own pain and the pain of others; and we can have competing pleasures (as a child my pleasure in pleasing my parents and my teachers can outstrip my pleasure in schoolwork, so I sacrifice my genuine interests for the love and approval of the grown-ups). Some pleasures don't make us happy, and some pains do.

'A people who conceive life to be the pursuit of happiness must be chronically unhappy,' wrote the anthropologist Marshall Sahlins. Whether or not this is true – and I think in many ways it is – it at least raises the question of why happiness should matter to us at

all. And why, more topically, there should have been
so many books published recently about happiness;
and why, indeed, the conference I have written this
essay for is entitled 'Should School Make You Happy?'
rather than, say, 'Should School make You Kind?', or
should school make you just or good, or even educated? Discussions of what makes a good life, and
whether virtue (or anything else) can be taught, are as
old as literate human inquiry. But happiness is now the
thing, and so we need to have some idea of what the
pursuit of happiness is the pursuit of; whether school
can make people anything (that is, how influenceable
are children, and in what ways); and what the much-
cherished phrase 'making someone happy' might
mean, and might mean now. And I think we should
bear in mind at the outset a few obvious salient truths.
First, that cruelty makes some people happy, and makes
most people happy at least some of the time. Second,
it is not clear that the pursuit of happiness, as seen in
the wider culture, necessarily brings out the best in
people; people can do terrible things as a means to the
end when that end is happiness. Indeed, the pursuit of
happiness can make people very unhappy. And third,
and most obvious, what makes people happy is often
very idiosyncratic, very personal and sometimes private. 'Happiness,' as Freud wrote, 'is something essentially subjective.' School, of course, might help people
find what makes them happy, but in this sense – and I
will come back to this – it can't make people happy.

Insofar as happiness is subjective – that what makes us happy is a kind of key to our sense of ourselves – we don't need to define it. We don't need to tell people what they already know. But children, of course, are in the process of discovering for the first time, as it were, what makes them happy, or what happiness is for them. And for this, as for everything else, they are dependent on the adults who look after them, at least to begin with.

There is one fundamental experience that every parent has with their child, and that every school-teacher has with the children they teach, which is: you can't tell a child that they are not enjoying themselves, you can only tell them that they shouldn't be. Think of a young child gleefully pinching his younger sister, or the child peeing on the carpet. As adults we know that we can't tell someone that a joke isn't funny – we can only tell them that they shouldn't be amused. Children get pleasure from things that adults don't want them to get pleasure from. And this, at least, lets us be clear about one thing: if we believe that school should make children happy, what we mean is that school should make them happy in ways we, the adults, approve of. We adults are the owners of the acceptable definitions of happiness. We don't think school should make you happy about tormenting animals. As human creatures – and this is particularly vivid in school-age children – there are pleasures that make us happy which are unacceptable. And, of course, just to make the picture even more complicated, people can enjoy being, can want to be, unhappy. Talking about happiness at its worst can make us sound simple-minded; but it brings us up against all the difficult questions about pleasure,. and therefore about what we think children should be protected from, and why.

Various people have said in various ways, at various times, that the truly valuable thing about psychoanalysis is that it is the one place left in our culture where you can be, and be seen to be, wholeheartedly unhappy. And whatever this says about psychoanalysis it seems to me to be more of a comment about the extreme pressure we are under these days, and that we put our children under, to be happy; which also means not to be unhappy. And you only have to give this a moment's thought to realize that something quite strange is going on here: that the more terrible the things that happen in the world are, the more we are coerced into being or seeming or seeing ourselves as happy. But what would it mean, as an adult, to be happy after watching the news, say? Or, as a child, to be happy after learning in school about the history of the slave trade? If you need to be happy, and need those around you to be happy too – in the same way that alcoholics need everyone around them to drink – then what do you do with your unhappiness? If the problem of the alcoholic is sobriety (not drink) then the problem of the happiness addict is his misery.

It is unrealistic, I think – and by 'unrealistic' I mean it is a demand that cannot be met – to assume that if all goes well in a child's life he or she will be happy. Not because life is the kind of thing that doesn't make you happy; but because happiness is not something one can ask of a child. Children, I think, suffer – in a way that adults don't always realize – under the pressure their parents put on them to be happy, which is the pressure not to make their parents unhappy, or more unhappy than they already are. 'Be happy' can be a paradoxical injunction, like 'be spontaneous'; if you do it you are not doing it, and if you are not doing it you are doing it. And the worst-case scenario could be generations of children cheated of what they were educated to believe was their right to happiness. Should school demand happiness of the pupils, or should school make you happy if your family can't? All this is a roundabout way of making a plea, on the one hand, for children to be inspired by realistic ideals, if that is not a contradiction in terms. And, on the other hand, that one of the things we might talk about today is not only what makes children happy – and so what can schools do to foster this project – but also, what kind of demand does it make on the children, that school should make them happy, *and* on the teachers who will, in one way or another, be asked to deliver this happiness?

If the original question – the question in Plato – was: can virtue be taught? and our question is: can happiness be taught? – we might wonder what the difference is between school trying to make people good and school wanting to make people happy. One of the most obvious differences, as I alluded to before, is that being good doesn't always make children (or adults) happy. In other words, if school should make you happy, then it shouldn't necessarily make you good; happiness as an ideal, or an aim, or a goal, has to affect the child's morality. If school should make you happy, what kind of morality is it going to teach, both implicitly and explicitly, in the service of this ideal? If, for example, school should make you kind, it would not be too difficult for the adults, with a minimum of ordinary hypocrisy, to come up with a set of guidelines, definitions of what constitutes a kind act; and these would be means to an end. But what kind of guidelines would be provided to help children be happy, given that happiness is, as Freud suggests, subjective, and that moral goodness does not always make the child happy (being good makes the child feel safe, that is, loved by those he needs, but not necessarily very alive)? What is the morality if happiness is the aim? Might the school be saying to the child: do only the things that really interest you, that really make you feel alive, whatever other people think? Would the school have to say the para-doxical thing: our rules are made to be broken because we know that, at least for some of you, only trans-gression and/or risk will make you feel fully alive, and for some of you feeling that kind of aliveness is the only authentic happiness. In promoting happiness in school, we would be promoting, at least for some of the pupils, excitement rather than safety. We would be saying – and this, of course, might be a good thing – don't avoid situations that might make you feel guilty, but learn to bear guilt.

It is not that promoting happiness at school in and of itself promotes risk; but it confronts the adults with the perennial question of whether, and in what situations, children might prefer safety to excitement, or vice versa. Because some children's happiness, at least some of the time, will reside in safety and other children's happiness will reside in excitement. And this will change at different stages in their lives. One of the main reasons that schools should offer up happiness as an ideal – whether or not school can make children happy – is that it gives the children, and their teachers, a more morally complex vision. Because adults cannot know beforehand what will make a child happy, they will be unable to construct and impose a morality that will make the children happy. It would be good to start our morality-making from seeing what makes people happy, rather than as a way of pre-empting them from finding out.

The pro-happiness school, at its best, will be a pro-moral improvisation school. This will put a heavy, but potentially interesting, burden on the teachers. Happiness may be good as an ideal because it changes our views about morality; it allows children in school to have a more intriguing and exciting version of what morality might involve. But happiness as a moral demand – you must be happy, and you are failing if you are not – is pernicious. If the pressure to be happy is disabling – what is the child under pressure to be happy going to do with her unhappiness? – the opportunity to be happy or, rather, to find what makes you happy, can only be a good thing. And yet, as we can't help but notice, taking opportunities for happiness can be, for both children and adults, morally complicated, and can also involve some unhappiness (think of the child in school preferring one friend over another, or wanting to study subjects of which her parents disapprove). So it seems to me that one thing education can do is help children find a language that can do justice to the pleasures and problems that happiness involves. So if I can just rephrase the title of this essay again, it might be, 'Should Education Make You Interested in Happiness?', and my answer would be yes. Should education make us happy? Well, no, but only because nothing and no one can make us happy, as in do something to us that will create this wonderful thing. What it can do is create the conditions in which children might be happy, and an environment in which they can begin to get a sense of the conflicts that happiness embroils them in. If, as John Lennon said, life is what happens to you when you are doing something else, then so, perhaps, is happiness.

One of the reasons I assume that we think education – or anything else, like parenting or good looks or money – should or could make us happy is because we are all too aware of what makes us unhappy. And we assume that if we take the unhappy-making thing out of the picture, our innate happiness will be there, waiting to happen. If we take the bully out of the class, the bullied will be happy; if I give up maths, which I hate, I will be happy. In other words, we can't use a version of logical common sense when it comes to happiness. It is better, indeed essential, that the bullying stops; but that, in and of itself, may or may not create the expected happiness. The bullied child, for example, may miss being punished by the bully and seek punishment elsewhere; or she may miss the intensity of the attention she gets from the bully. And, of course, she may be relieved and happier. Schools, clearly, should do everything they can to diminish all those things that are known to make children unhappy – elitism, bullying, excessive emphasis on competition instead of collaboration, boring and/or humiliating teaching, covert or explicit sexism or racism, and so on. But I think it needs to be acknowledged that doing this can be, at least for some children, simply creating the preconditions in which they might find what makes them happy. What Philip Larkin called in his poem 'Born Yesterday' 'a skilled,/ Vigilant, flexible, Unemphasised, enthralled/ Catching of happiness' can't be arranged or engineered for each individual child. Without these good-enough conditions, which are hard enough to create, it is very difficult for the individual child to pursue her happiness; but with them, there can be no guarantee that her happiness will be there for the taking. And this is why I think it is useful to think in terms of the child's official and unofficial development; and to think of schools as double-agents, places that sponsor the good, nice person and the strange, eccentric delinquent that each child is. The good citizen pretending to himself or herself that he or she is not a furtive criminal, and the furtive criminal pretending to himself or herself that he or she is not a good citizen, is not a recipe for the possibility of happiness. Unbearable choices make impossible lives.

The most important thing about school for the child is that it is not the family; it is another place (as it is, of course, also for the teachers). The so-called mental health professions often want to say that whether or not education should make you happy, it can't make you happy if your home doesn't, or if, more fatefully, you were born temperamentally unhappy. No one could, or should, now underestimate the significance of parents and siblings in a child's life; but nor should this be used to obscure just what school can do for children (think how life-changing certain teachers have been for many people). Nothing in the child's life will make her more unhappy than her family, or its absence; and a considerable amount of children's unhappiness in school is bound up with their family life. Every teacher knows that teaching is never just the conveying of information, but rather a way of joining, at a distance, the families of all the children they teach.

But because school is also another place – and no one should underestimate the challenge for a child to go from the closed world of the family to the open road of school – it provides the possibility for new forms of happiness. Most of us remember as children going to visit other children's families and noticing, with varying degrees of exhilaration and dread, that they did things differently there. And this is more true of school because a school is not even a family, the only social group the child has previously known. School, whatever else it is, is the place where the child can find both new ideas about happiness, and notice new ways of being happy. One of the most extraordinary things about other people, insofar as they exist for us, are the ways in which they can be happy. The child, given half a chance, can't help but notice, from other children and from the teachers, that there are many kinds of good life. They may even come across people at school they admire who don't think happiness is very important, who believe, as the American literary critic Lionel Trilling did, that no morally serious person could be interested in happiness. So should education make you happy? It should at least show you the forms that happiness can take, and which you can't get from your family. The trouble with one's family is that that is all they are.

We should, of course, be wary of people who are keen to tell us that suffering is good for us; all suffering, it seems to me, is bad, although some suffering is inevitable. But that doesn't mean that we shouldn't also be alert when we are promoting happiness, something that seems at first glance so self-evidently a good thing. Words and phrases like 'happiness', 'well-being', 'flourishing' and 'fulfilling potential' all make us feel better; and no one in their right minds would want school to make children unhappy, or stop them fulfilling their potential, or persuade them that life wasn't worth living (something the adults around them will feel sometimes, even if they would prefer not to).

So let us ask: what is being promoted in the name of happiness and that means both what happiness is, and what happiness might be a cover-story for? And what might the pursuit of happiness – in education and elsewhere – be distracting us from? If education should make you happy, what will have to be sacrificed in its pursuit? Can an adult who has a realistic sense of contemporary life be happy now? And if she can, what does she need not to notice and to feel in order to sustain her happiness? We might, for example, want school-age children to have a capacity for happiness, an openness to it, a fearlessness with regard to it, but not an addiction to it. Do we really want our children to believe that only a happy life is a good life? How many of the people we admire from the past were happy? Because if happiness is pursued at all costs, the cost will be too great. We may end up by saying something like: education should be showing children good ways of bearing their unhappiness, and good ways of taking their happiness when it comes.

Happiness is a very difficult thing to be clear about; and especially the happiness of children. We don't, for example, want to burden our children with having to be happy because we can't be, and because if they are happy we parents and teachers can feel better about ourselves; which casts our children as anti-depressants (parents are more dependent on their children than their children are on them). And we are all struck by children's capacity for pleasure, how much they can relish being alive, how happy they often seem to be, as we say, by nature. But I think we need to distinguish, as far as we can, most children's innate appetite for life from the adults' need, the adults' demand, that they, the children, be happy. The philosopher Alasdair MacIntyre writes that according to the utilitarian principle, when people choose to do things with a view to promoting the greatest happiness for the greatest number, 'it is always necessary to ask what actual project or purpose is being concealed by its use'. As though, he implies, when people do things to make people happy they are likely to be, at best, doing many other things as well, and, at worst, concealing what they are actually doing. Indeed MacIntyre seems to be suggesting that we should be particularly suspicious of the promoters of happiness; as though 'happiness' is an unusually good word to smuggle a whole lot of other things in under. As though anyone who thought education should make you happy was really thinking that education should make you a whole lot of other things that sound better if they are called happiness. Coca-Cola are promoting happiness, but they are actually selling drinks. I don't know whether I am as suspicious as MacIntyre is, but I do think we need to ask: if education should make you happy, what is it going to have to make you in order for you to be happy?

II Truancy Now

Psychoanalysis has had a lot of stories to tell about truant minds; indeed, it is the truancy of the so-called mind that psychoanalysis has attempted both to rein in and to contain, and to sponsor and to celebrate. When Freud wrote that the rider has to guide the horse in the direction the horse wants to go, or that the ego was not master in his own house, or talked about what are now called Freudian slips, or described people as the ambivalent animals, he was describing modern people as being riven with intentions and counter-intentions. For Freud it was not that there were truant minds, but that the mind was truant; that when people act in their own best interests they don't always know what their best interests are, or whether their best interests are the things that actually matter most to them; or, indeed, what their interests are. Because what we desire is forbidden to us, in Freud's view, we have to work hard not to know what it is; if we are asked what we are working on, we can say that we are working on our ignorance. If we speak in Freud's language, the ego is the part of ourselves that wants safety and survival, and the id is the part of ourselves that wants sensual satisfaction whatever the cost. To put it slightly differently, there is a part of ourselves that has no interest in our best interests, if our best interests are taken to be our own survival. It is not that a part of ourselves prefers risk to safety, it is that a part of ourselves doesn't use this vocabulary; it is not that a part of ourselves is self-destructive, it is that a part of ourselves has no regard for whether our actions are destructive or construct-ive. Indeed, the whole notion of self-destructive behaviour presumes to know not merely what con-structive behaviour is, but what the person most wants (what, at their best, they most want).

Adults who look after pre-adolescent children have to know, have to have some sense of, what is in the child's best interests. They are in this sense the guardians of the children's future or potential selves. The very small child doesn't know he mustn't touch the hot cup; the older child may try out touching the hot cup, to find out for himself, to learn from experi-ence. The truant mind of the truant child is experi-menting: he is finding out whether the cup is hot, that is, whether the adult's words can be trusted (whether the adult's words matter to him); whether the adult is keeping an eye on him; whether he can withstand the adult's punishment or even hatred. You find out what the rules are made of by trying to break them; to begin with you learn what it is to fol-low a rule; and then you find out what can be done with the whole business of following rules; what it is about rule-following that is satisfying, and who it is you are satisfying by following the rules. St Paul talks famously in the Epistle to the Romans about how the law entered human history 'to increase the trespass'; that 'where there is no law there is no transgression'; and that 'through the law comes knowledge of sin'. It is not simply that rules are made to be broken, but that the rules tell you that there is something to break. If there was no law it would be impossible to transgress. The rules, whatever else they might be, are an invitation to find out what rules are; which means to find out what kind of person you are. Even though by being born into a society we consent to its rules, there is never a moment when we, as it were, sit down and consent to them. Adolescence is the time in people's lives when they begin to notice that there are other things you can do with the rules than be spellbound by them. The adolescent is somebody who is trying to get himself kidnapped from a cult.

In our ordinary everyday use of the term a 'truant' is someone who stays away from school, as *Chambers English Dictionary* says quaintly, 'without leave or good reason'; people play truant as though it were a game and, by implication, as though it were something that comes to an end. But in its older and now obsolete meaning a 'truant' is a 'vagrant' or an 'idler'; all the meanings want us to picture the truant as someone who takes time out of work. When Hamlet asks Horatio in Act 1 why he has come back from Wittenberg, Horatio replies, 'A truant disposition, good my lord'; to which Hamlet responds, 'I would not hear your enemy say so.' Hamlet cannot possibly accept this description of his friend, which he calls 'your own report/ Against yourself: I know you are no truant.' Hamlet so objects because a truant, in his view, is a terrible thing to call oneself. He accuses Horatio of self-betrayal, of siding with his enemy against himself. By calling himself a truant Horatio has taken time out from the work of giving an accurate account of oneself. We tend to think of people playing truant from school, from some external, often institutional, constraint; such as being on day release, or taking a holiday from one's real responsibilities. What Hamlet reminds us of is that it is possible to play truant with oneself. Freud says we can't help but do this, while Hamlet says we *shouldn't* do this. And all this brings me to the simple point that the adolescent is the person who needs to experiment with self-betrayal; is the person who needs to find out what it is, or what it might be, to betray oneself. Which is not what it means to break the rules, but what it means to break the rules that are of special, of essential, value to oneself. And in order to do this you have to find out what these rules are. So-called delinquent behaviour is the unconscious attempt to find the rules that really matter to the individual. And this is one of the most – if not *the* most – frightening quests.

Betraying other people matters only if in so doing one has betrayed oneself. This is what truant minds are for, and this is what adolescence ineluctably embroils modern people in: the attempt to find out

what it is to betray oneself, and what the consequences of self-betrayal are. 'I have always admired
people who have left behind them an incomprehensible mess,' Bob Dylan once said in an interview. The
psychoanalyst D. W. Winnicott talks about what he
calls delinquent children having to 'test the environment' through really bad behaviour. Children, for
example, who had been evacuated from their homes
during the war had to be able to be difficult when
they finally got home just to ensure that their parents
could be trusted not to send them away again. Only
by being really difficult can the child discover whether
the parents are worth having; whether they are resili-
ent and robust. If the child, the adolescent and the
adult are never really difficult they never find out
what the world and themselves are really like. It is as
if we are involved in a continual love test with the
world, trying to find out whether we and it are worth
wanting, worth loving. Being truant minds, having
what Horatio and Freud call a 'truant disposition', is,
I think, a part of this testing, this experimenting,
that begins in adolescence and, if things go wrong, is
given up on in adolescence. But the adolescents who
give up on this fundamental project in adolescence
may turn into adults who secretly envy adolescents;
who believe that adolescents are having the best kinds
of life available.

The Authenticity Issue

For Carole Tulloch

Great outpourings of expressive feeling are not relevant
to making art. Much more so is the both simple and
complex fact of how you group things together.

Briony Fer, *Eva Hesse: Studiowork*

Just as there are phantom limbs there are phantom
histories, histories that are severed and discarded, but
linger on as thwarted possibilities and compelling nos-
talgias. After the amputation we live as if, it feels as if,
the limb is still there. Its loss is known, even mourned,
but it is still experienced as somehow present; it is a
loss at once acknowledged and invisible. We live a
double life, a doublethink in relation to this absence.
Like Freud's account of fetishism in which 'only one
current' in a person's life had not recognized the disturbing fact of there being two sexes, while 'another
current took full account of the fact', the two states of
mind 'existing side by side', the phantom history is
known and not known at the same time. It lives on as
a strange kind of unfinished and unfinishable business.
And this is particularly vivid when a word changes or

loses its meaning over time, when its meaning becomes ironized, or turned into its opposite, when 'wicked', for example, is used to mean 'brilliant' instead of 'evil' in the old-fashioned sense, or when 'nice' comes to mean 'pleasant' rather than 'accurate'.

'Authenticity', I think, is an unusually interesting example of the phantom-limb effect – a significant casualty of ironization – because the tone in which it is used has changed remarkably quickly. Where once it referred to the most valuable of essences, it is now all too easily used to say that there is no such thing – that, for example, one's authentic self is one role or version of the self among many others, perhaps even a preferred one, but one merely rhetorically privileged by being called authentic; or that to search for the authentic text of *Hamlet* is to misunderstand, to fail to historicize, the working practices of Renaissance drama. The whole idea of authenticity is generally regarded as a misleading or even pernicious concept, the last and peculiarly modern bastion of a now discredited essentialism. Where once we might have asked whether something, say, a work of art, was authentic, now we might just want an account of what is good about it. Where once we might have been unsettled about whether someone was authentic, now we might ask, more pragmatically, what are they trying to do, what do they want or want to communicate, by being like that? I think we are, however, freer now not to care about the authenticity of objects than about the authenticity of people; forgeries can dismay or intrigue us, but people we experience as phoneys are more radically disturbing. Inauthentic objects can cost us money, inauthentic people can cost us a lot more. People we call inauthentic can frighten us, whereas inauthentic objects do not, and it is worth wondering why this might be. The obvious answer is that an inauthentic person might harm us, that we may be confounded or exploited by them, that we can't be sure what they are up to; and yet the reasons we think this way are themselves revealing. Why, for example, might we assume that an authentic person isn't dangerous? The distinction between the authenticity of objects and the authenticity of people is one worth bearing in mind. But for the moment I want to consider the idea of an authentic history, and what an authentic history of the notion of authenticity might be. Could there be a contemporary version, an update, say, of Lionel Trilling's great book *Sincerity and Authenticity*, and what would it be like?

The phantom-limb effect — an absence acknowledged through an apparent presence — is clearly at work in the idea of authenticity. The culture I grew up in informed me that I had an authentic, true self; and then I discovered in my adolescence in the 1960s and early 1970s that there was no such thing. I continued to live as if I had one, but the more I looked for it, and tried to feel its presence, the more I realized it wasn't there. But having it removed made it real in a new way; its absence gave me room to think about it, whereas its presence had been pre-emptive. Before its amputation, I could wonder what my authentic self was, and aspire to it; afterwards, I could wonder what I was, what was possible, if there was no such thing. And later, as a psychoanalyst, I could wonder what calling instinctual life 'authentic' added to the conversation; I could wonder why thinking about authenticity seemed itself to be an authentic thing to do. I would now say that all the prescribed aims of psychoanalysis – instinctual gratification, becoming one's true self, becoming the subject of one's desire, and so on – are, inevitably, all attempts at achieving authenticity, even if psychoanalysts would not describe those aims as such. The phantom-limb effect fades; but 'authenticity' is a difficult word to give up, or more difficult than it seems. And this, in itself, is of interest. It still gives us something to talk about. So I want to consider, briefly, two things. First, what do we lose if we drop it from our vocabulary, and what kind of gain might this be? And second, what might have happened, and be happening, to its usage? When does it seem to be the right word, and when it is the right word, what is right about it? The three examples I want to use to show how the notion of authenticity can be worked are not from any kind of research but just from recent reading.

★

The poet John Clare, in the early nineteenth century, writes about his childhood reading: 'from the sixpenny Romances of "Cinderella", "Little Red Riding Hood", "Jack and the Beanstalk", "Zig-zag", "Prince Cherry", etc., etc., and great was the pleasure, pain or surprise increased by allowing them authenticity, for I firmly believed every page I read'.

Clare, the so-called 'peasant poet', was greatly exercised by his authenticity as a poet. In this piece of autobiography, he makes some interesting links, and strikingly talks of authenticity as something allowed, as in allowed for and given permission. When the young Clare allows these romances authenticity, they have a much more immediate and powerful effect on him; 'great was the pleasure, pain or surprise increased by allowing them authenticity, for I firmly believed every page I read'. So, not to allow authenticity would be to hold these stories at a distance, to diminish their emotional impact. Clare's implied logic is that only if he allows these romances authenticity can he believe them, and only if he believes them can he be sufficiently moved by them. Allowing authenticity – which means something like suspending doubt – allows Clare to become absorbed in these particular works of art, and this enables him to feel what he feels.

The implications here are twofold: not to allow authenticity is to defend yourself against the impact of the work and the sheer scale of your own feelings.

It is as if Clare is wondering what the preconditions
are for contact, for exchange, for immediacy, and the
answer is, the allowing of authenticity. Not allowing
the stories to be real means not allowing them to
have an effect. Authenticity, Clare acknowledges, is
something that is conferred; you can ascribe it to
something or you can withhold it; as though it were
an attitude of mind, an approach towards rather than
an ingredient of an object. Clare knows that the
romances might not be true, but by treating them as
though they are, he makes them live for him. Here
Clare is alive to the loss involved in not allowing
them authenticity. If you treat a work of literary art
as authentic, it brings out the best in you because you
get the best out of it. But it is nevertheless a para-
doxical claim; you must treat them as if they are
authentic. If we find it increasingly difficult to believe
in authenticity, we can believe in 'as-if authenticity',
the suspension of disbelief. Clare suggests, though
he wouldn't have put it like this, that we need to hold
on to what happens when we treat stories – and perhaps people – as if they are authentic. Whatever the
authentic was, it gave us access to the other thing we
value most, intense feeling and surprise. Allowing the
authenticity of the object is a cure for our own illusions
of omniscience. If we don't allow the object authenticity, we don't allow ourselves an emotional life, the
full range of our feelings. We don't have to believe in
authenticity, we just have to remember and believe in

what we thought authenticity was like. Clare is saying that what we value most about ourselves – pleasure, pain and surprise – is made possible by our belief in authenticity. When we no longer allow authenticity we will be quite different creatures, creatures for whom pleasure, pain and surprise are no longer the supreme values, the privileged experiences. Clare, I think, had some dark (and possibly well-justified) forebodings about this.

John Banville's great novel *The Newton Letter* (1982) is the story of an academic who rents a house in the Irish countryside to finish a book he is writing about Newton, and finds all his plans waylaid. He finds himself having a sexual relationship with one woman from a nearby house while falling in love with another woman who lives in the house he is renting. In this maelstrom, he discovers new versions of himself and begins to see different versions of each of the women. Were we all, the narrator asks, 'dividing thus and multiplying like amoebas? In this spawning of multiple selves I seemed to see the awesome force of my love, which in turn served to convince me anew of its authenticity.'

Once again – and this is characteristic, I think, of its modern usage – the idea of authenticity is trailed by an irony. If for Clare the authentic has become that seeming contradiction in terms, the 'as-if authentic', so for Banville the sign of his own authenticity, of the authenticity of his love, is that he and his women become, as it were, multiple personalities. The authenticity resides not in any one of them – the narrator is not asking which is the real me, or the real woman – but in the fact that the old idea of authenticity goes out the window. What is authentic now is that you can't tell, indeed might not even be interested in, which version of the self is authentic. The authentic is not the true or the real or the fundamental; it is the relinquishing of such possibilities: it is the entire repertoire. You know your love is authentic when it produces new versions of yourself and the beloved, none of which is more real than any other. And it is worth noting that Banville, in his sly way, runs together two vocabularies in the narrator's description of his authenticity: the old quasi-religious vocabulary of 'the awesome force of my love' with the new secular scientific language of 'amoebas'. (Not 'go forth and multiply', but 'divide and multiply'.) The only authenticity available to the modern subject, we are now insistently told, is the authenticity of his dividedness. Unity and consensus – in the self and outside the self – is replaced by conflict and co-existence. From Banville's view, love doesn't bring us together, as it used to, it splits us up. For the narrator here it is authentic to have no essence; multiplicity and disarray are the real thing. Banville's narrator, in this sense, abides by Gertrude Stein's famous modernist injunction in *Tender Buttons*: 'Act so that there is no use in a center.' But for Banville's narrator this is no longer an experiment or a strategy, but an inevitability. It is authentic to acknowledge that there is no centre, so the word undoes itself. Banville's narrator, in other words, wants to have it both ways: he wants to hold on to authenticity, but by letting the word betray itself; you know your love is authentic when it multiplies you and the beloved, but what makes it real is that you cannot identify any of these selves as more real or authentic than any other. Your authenticity resides in your acknowledgement that the real, the authentic, the centre, can no longer be located. You have a measure that shows you that there is no longer anything to measure. Real love makes us unreal to ourselves and to others, and by the same token makes others unreal to us. We are relieved of the burden of judgement, but not, of course, of the burden of preference. We may not be able to locate an authentic version of ourselves, but there are some we like more than others. But, at least in love, we are helpless bystanders. There is a show going on and it is ourselves. And we can't use a word like 'authenticity' to tell us what matters, or what matters most.

Once again, the authentic is being linked with the strongest forms of feeling, as though the idea of authenticity is somehow bound up with keeping our passions alive. Indeed, we may be tempted – even those of us who don't 'believe' in authenticity – to conclude that our passionate selves are our most authentic selves. If we were to drop authenticity from our vocabulary, we may have to drop the picture of ourselves as passionate creatures, albeit troubled by our passions; and this might be the draw and the dread of the enemies of authenticity. That once we lose authenticity, so much else will be lost with it. The collapse of authenticity would bring in its wake proliferating redescriptions not of what we are really like – which would be like replacing belief in God with belief in something else equally demanding – but of what? We have to imagine the as-yet unimaginable: a world without grails. A world in which the difficulty is not recognizing and locating the desired and elusive object, but giving up on a world of such objects. The 'awesome force' of the narrator's love in *The Newton Letter* is a force for radical disorientation that ushers in the acknowledgement that there is no orientation available. 'I will show you fear in a handful of specialists,' the poet John Ashbery writes in *Flow Chart*.

In her new memoir *Room for Doubt,* the American writer Wendy Lesser has a chapter about living in Berlin; and her sense of what contemporary Berlin is like prompts invidious comparison with New York. There is, she has a sense, 'a richly inflected innocence' about contemporary Berlin,

> a zeal for the new that is both premised on appreci-
> ation of and wariness about the old. We have noth-
> ing like it in America. Every few years New York

(and then the rest of the country) goes into a tortured soul-search and decides that we are all too ironic, that irony must now be thrown out so that something more – More what? More childlike? More authentic? More credulous? – something fresher and newer, at any rate, can be ushered in. But you cannot will such reforms.

The antidote for irony, and its supposedly enervating effect, is, in Lesser's telling list, something more childlike, more authentic, more credulous; reminiscent of Clare, and Banville in a different way, when the word 'authenticity' is used, it conveys something about immediacy. Irony is, as we say, a distance regulator and there is something that we nostalgic Romantics feel estranged from and want to get back to or closer to: the childlike, the authentic, states of credulity. The authentic in this list represents the retreat of scepticism, doubt, even reflection. It is trustworthy, and we can entrust ourselves to it. It allows us to yield rather than requiring our vigilance. If we can be more childlike, authentic and credulous, it is assumed, something fresher and newer can be ushered in, as though irony is our defence against the new, a kind of character armour, and if we could shrug it off, we could be more vulnerable, more receptive, capable of exchange and not ambitious for insulation. The authentic, in Lesser's sentence, refers to all that we are not; we could say that it does useful work as a way of

imagining precisely all that we feel most urgently
lacking. But for Lesser this is a false lure, as though
authenticity is about recapturing an innocence that
never existed, or can't exist again; as though the desire
for authenticity, like the desire to be childlike or
credulous, is a failure to mourn, an inability to grow
up and out of such vague and insubstantial longings.
Berlin is keen for the new, and appreciative but wary
of the old; authenticity, as a modern aspiration, is
regressive, as in, say, fascist ideology; it prefers, Lesser
implies, the (mythical) old, and cannot properly appre-
ciate the old because it cannot afford to be wary. This,
at least, is what Lesser intimates, in her reflections on
Berlin, since credulity and authenticity characterize
the Nazi way. Authenticity, in this context, smacks
of the unspeakable cruelty people are capable of when
they are sufficiently credulous to act on behalf of an
absolute truth. Once you allow this version of authenticity – or once you face the fact that to be childlike is
also to be vicious and not merely sweet, and to be
credulous is to be manipulable and manipulative –
you cultivate the darker side of the so-called passionate self.

These are three usages, three versions of authenticity.
Clare's 'as-if authenticity', once allowed, ushers in the
passionate, surprised and surprising self. Banville's narrator's authentic love multiplies selves and, by rendering
each of the selves equally authentic, makes multiplicity

itself the only authenticity available; this authenticity ushers in the plural self, helplessly proliferating, unable to sort itself out; 'authentic', in this case, means the disarray that happens to happen. And then there is Lesser's unself-ironizing, credulous and childlike authenticity, complicit with fascism, and averse to irony. Only Clare, you will notice, has a good word for the passionate self, and he promotes not authenticity itself, but the allowance of it; he treats it as a useful fiction but perhaps a dangerous myth. For Banville's narrator the authentic is not something aspired to as myth or fiction, it is just the music, or the noise, of what happens; love is authentic when it makes your own and the beloved's authenticity indiscernible. That is what love does, it cures us of our belief in authenticity, as though the idea of authenticity is something we use to protect ourselves from love. For Lesser, irony is preferred because it tempers the immediacy, the brutality, of passion. In their different ways, each of them is asking what the idea of authenticity allows us to hold on to. What does the desire for authenticity help us to forget? What are we fearful of losing if the word is ironized out of contention? Or, to put it another way, what can you be for if you are against authenticity? Once, that is, authenticity has been taken away from you. The point about authenticity is that we once thought we could have it, not that it does or doesn't exist.

Negative Capabilities

What's past help, should be past grief.

Shakespeare, *The Winter's Tale*

reason's no
better off than its ambience . . .

A. R. Ammons, 'Hibernaculum'

I The Horse

When Freud, in the *New Introductory Lectures*, describes the relationship between the ego and the id as similar to the relationship between a rider and his horse, we have the feeling that Freud is bending over backwards to make psychoanalysis accessible; as though the radical redescriptions of psychoanalysis are entirely conventional, utterly familiar to us. And yet Freud renders the conventional image absurd; he invites us to imagine a world in which the horse is in charge, and in which the rider is involved in a kind of pretence. It is a picture of two creatures who do not speak the same language, but one of them is pretending that they do:

> The horse supplies the locomotive energy, while the rider has the privilege of deciding on the goal and of guiding the powerful animal's movement. But only too often there arises between the ego and the id the not precisely ideal situation of the rider being obliged to guide the horse along the path by which it itself wants to go.

We begin on a familiar path – 'the rider has the privilege of deciding ...' – but the writer guides us in the direction that the horse wants to go. In this 'not precisely ideal situation', which indeed makes a mockery of our ideals of purpose, of progress, of autonomy, there is direction but not for us. The rider is at once masterful – he looks masterful, as the great portraits of the mounted kings and emperors suggest – and helpless, competent but fundamentally incapable. Where then, Freud wants us to ask, does our competence reside, what is our skill or our talent, what can we do if the rider is too often obliged to guide the horse along the path it wants to go in? And Freud's answer is very simple: the competence of the ego is in its capacity to defend itself; and to defend itself, above all, as Freud's image of the rider and his horse intimates, from the knowledge of this helplessness. Like all simple answers this has complicated consequences.

When Freud wrote in *Beyond the Pleasure Principle* that 'protection against stimuli is an almost more important function for the living organism than reception of stimuli', he was making it very clear that as receptive creatures we are helpless, but as self-protective creatures we have at least the illusion of some kind of power and freedom (the rider has found a way of making himself feel powerful on his horse). 'Almost more important,' of course, suggests a doubt in Freud's mind, but the phrase 'choice of neurosis', for example, emphasizes the point. Psychoanalysis, whatever else it is, is a story about how we protect ourselves from our helplessness, from our incapacities; from our knowledge of these things and from our experience of them. Sexuality, as taboo, is exciting; helplessness is not. Psychoanalysis has tried, as it were, to make the case for sexuality; it has never been able to make the case for helplessness. 'What one finds problematic,' the philosopher Richard Rorty writes, in *Philosophical Papers*, 'is a function of what one thinks important.' Helplessness has been at once both the abiding preoccupation of psychoanalysis and, perhaps unsurprisingly, a preoccupation resistant to articulation. The choice, if that is what it is, between the ego-psychologies and the anti-ego-psychologies is a choice between descriptions of the form and function of helplessness in the fate of the modern human subject. It is not sexuality that has been the contentious, the divisive, issue in psychoanalysis after Freud, it is resourcelessness.

As Strachey wrote in his illuminating editorial introduction to Freud's *Inhibitions, Symptoms and Anxiety*,
once trauma is the issue, helplessness is the heart of
the matter, whether we are talking of the trauma of
desire or the trauma of object loss. If helplessness is
fundamentally what we defend ourselves against it is
not surprising that the ways we have of doing this
make us feel powerful; our sense of power is a function of our helplessness, our games of autonomy are
our self-cure for resourcelessness. 'The fundamental
determinant of automatic anxiety,' Strachey writes,

> is the occurrence of a traumatic situation; and the
> essence of this is an experience of helplessness on
> the part of the ego in the face of an accumulation of
> excitation ... the various specific dangers which are
> liable to precipitate a traumatic situation at different
> times of life. These are briefly: birth, loss of the mother
> as an object, loss of the penis, loss of the object's love,
> loss of the super-ego's love.

Our lives are always threatening to be too much for
us; what Strachey calls 'the accumulation of excitation' is what renders us helpless. In this picture we are
always at risk of being overwhelmed by ourselves; our
helplessness is our inability to master, to bind, to bear
(to represent) this excitation. In this ongoing crisis of
overexcitement, at least in this picture, our helplessness is so obviously the problem that it cannot be seen

as the solution to anything. It is starkly what we need to defend ourselves from. In psychoanalytic language we might say that we have lost our ambivalence about our helplessness; it is described now only as something we hate, not as something we could ever love. It is, indeed, problematic because it is so important.

Anna Freud writes of what she calls the 'constructive' trauma of helplessness: 'it is the painful experience of helplessness when confronted with powerful stimulation which induces the child's ego gradually to learn to exercise and to assume the functions of the stimulus barrier'. At its best, she suggests, helplessness makes the ego stronger, more able to 'exercise and assume the functions of the protective shield'. But also, at its worst, helplessness makes the ego stronger, more imperious, more prone to triumphalism (to the triumphalism of fascism, say, or the dogmatic certainties of religious fundamentalisms). If it might seem naive to write in praise of our helplessness it is surely worth wondering, from a psychoanalytic point of view, why we experience it as a fatal flaw. Or, to put it slightly differently, why it is so difficult, in secular language, to describe our helplessness as a gift as well as a curse. So much seems to depend on what our helplessness inspires in us.

II The Helpless

I

We should
Never dare offer our helplessness as a good
Bargain, without at least
Promising to overcome a misfortune we blame
History or Banks or the weather for: but this beast
Dares to exist without shame.

W. H. Auden, 'Mundus et Infans'

'I am myself alone,' Richard Duke of Gloucester —
the future Richard III — boasts towards the end of
the third part of Shakespeare's *Henry VI*. He is both
by himself and only himself, uninformed by others.
He lives, as we say, as a law unto himself; as a man
who, in the words of Lady Anne, who he will later
court, 'know'st no law of God nor man'. There is in
Richard a pretence of exemption, a supposed freedom from inevitable involvements and obligation,
summed up by one of his accusers, Queen Elizabeth:
'Thy self is self-misused,' she says, to which Richard
replies, 'Why then, by God — '. To say 'I am myself
alone' acknowledges that one needs a world to be
alone in. Richard was also living, as he can't help

but acknowledge, in what we have come to call an enchanted world, a world of spirits and demons, and indeed of God. There was a limit set to how self-sufficient, to how alone, he could claim to be. Even in disavowing his bond with others, as he does consistently throughout the play, he recognizes that such bonds exist. 'Conscience is but a word that cowards use,' he suggests, using the word himself in a covert admission of his own cowardice, and of what we might think of as a disavowed part of himself – he has registered the word, but only as a word, and only as a word used by others. 'I am myself alone,' as a boast rather than a plaint, is a description of what Richard thinks he has been able to dispense with: the need of, the regard of (and for), other people. It is the claim of a character one critic has called 'a sardonic narcissist'; the sardonic are, in the words of *The Oxford English Dictionary*, 'bitter, scornful, mocking'.

'The hell of the narcissist,' the French analyst Serge Viderman wrote, 'is the tyranny of his need for others.' As though there is something disabling about the need for other people. At its most minimal the need for other people exposes one's own frustration; it exposes to oneself and to others those things without which one cannot live, but that one cannot provide for oneself. To be able to feel one's frustration – in actuality an unusually difficult thing to do – requires a measure of helplessness; and Richard, we can say – and this is part of his uncanny allure both for the audience and for the other characters – implicitly but consistently ablates his own helplessness until the very end of the play. His language about himself, in all its tortuous and subtle dissimulation, insists on his own invulnerability; or rather, it is an attempt at invulnerability (which is always linked with sadism: I am invulnerable only because you are vulnerable). So it is of interest, I think, that one of Shakespeare's three uses of the word 'helpless' is in *Richard III* (the other two are in *The Comedy of Errors*); the first use of 'helplessness' cited by *The Oxford English Dictionary* is 1731, and it is, I imagine, of some significance that the word becomes currency in the eighteenth century.

The word 'helpless' is used early in the first act of *Richard III* by Lady Anne as she is brought the dead body of her father-in-law, King Henry VI. The man who within the space of the play will become (illegitimately) Richard III has already murdered, among many others, her husband and his father, and will eventually court her and have her killed. He feels like an implacable force – is indeed often referred to in the play as a, or the, devil – and renders people around him, especially the women, helpless. But at this moment in the play Lady Anne is faced with the king's body, and the impending catastrophe. Looking at his wounded body, and weeping, she says: 'Lo, in these windows that let forth thy life/ I pour the helpless balm of my poor eyes.' She is helplessly crying, but her tears, the 'helpless balm', can't help the dead king or herself. What she can't help but express, the tears she is shedding, are no help. Her helplessness is no help to her (it is, of course, a familiar topos that helplessness can't be helped, and is no help; consider Beckett's *Ill Seen, Ill Said*: 'She sits on, erect and rigid, in the deepening gloom. Such helplessness to move she cannot help').

The ineffectuality of tears is a continual theme. The play is full of references to tears as both impotent and easily feigned; as though grief should also make us suspicious. In this case Anne's tears can neither bring the king back to life, nor stem the evil that is Richard. Nothing can make her tears helpful balm; indeed 'helpless balm' is a contradiction in terms, because if it is helpless it is not balm at all. In this desperate scene nothing can be done: helplessness is tantamount to hopelessness. Lady Anne can refer to the king's dead body as a 'holy load'; but again to our modern or, rather, secular ears, it could be – as such scenes more obviously are in Shakespeare's later tragedies – in miniature, a scene of what we might be tempted to call 'catastrophic disillusionment', and which we have learned from Weber to call disenchantment: the acknowledgement that there is no (redemptive) magic within our power. This raises many questions: can we experience helplessness – can we notice that there may be such a thing as 'helpless balm' – without needing to re-enchant the world (that is to say, without talking of religious providentialism of

one kind or another, or now of the wonders of science
and technology, or indeed of art)? Can we acknowledge our helplessness and do without what Leo Ber-
sani has called 'the culture of redemption'? How has it
come about that something so fundamental to our being
as helplessness is akin, for us, to hopelessness? Richard,
we might think – and as Freud did think – enacted a
malign solution to his own helplessness. What would a
benign solution be? Why, to put it as starkly as possible,
does our helplessness so often tend to make us what we
call bad, or, at least, make us feel bad?

In 'Some Character-Types Met with in Psychoanalytic Work', Freud uses Richard III as his example of
what he calls 'the exceptions', those people whose
neuroses, Freud writes,

> were connected with some experience or suffering
> to which they had been subjected in their earliest
> childhood, one in respect of which they knew them-
> selves to be guiltless, and which they could look
> upon as an unjust disadvantage. The privileges they
> claimed as a result of this injustice and the rebel-
> liousness it engendered, had contributed not a little
> to intensify the conflicts leading to the outbreak of
> their neurosis.

The exceptions have suffered something they could
do nothing about, and have made a privilege of
necessity; they have been inspired, so to speak, by a

bad bout of helplessness. Richard, in his opening
soliloquy, says, as paraphrased by Freud:

> Nature has done me a grievous wrong in denying me
> the beauty of form which wins human love. Life owes
> me reparation for this, and I will see that I get it. I have
> a right to be an exception, to disregard the scruples by
> which others let themselves be held back. I may do
> wrong myself, since wrong has been done to me.

The exceptions, in Freud's examples, are not the
agents of their undoing; their victimhood becomes a
form of entitlement. For Richard it is, in a sense, an
opportunity to invent his own morality; or at least to
exempt himself from the morality of others. 'I, that
am curtail'd of this fair proportion,' he says in the
famous soliloquy, quoted by Freud,

> Cheated of feature by dissembling Nature,
> Deform'd, unfinish'd, sent before my time
> Into this breathing world, scarce half made up,
> And that so lamely and unfashionable,
> That dogs bark at me as I halt by them;

Freud, as we shall see, comes back to this stark
image of being 'sent before [our] time/ Into this
breathing world, scarce half made up' (Richard, Freud
remarks, 'is an enormous magnification of something
we find in ourselves as well'). It is an image of Rich-

ard's original helplessness; it is a predicament inflicted. Like Lady Anne's 'helpless balm' of tears, he couldn't help it happening to him, and this became, through his self-cure for it, no help for him or others. None of us choose our 'feature'. 'We all think we have reason to reproach Nature and our destiny for congenital and infantile disadvantages,' Freud writes by way of commentary in Richard's soliloquy: 'we all demand reparation for early wounds to our narcissism, our self-love'. Freud, as we shall also see, turns this fundamental situation – what we make out of our original helplessness – into an explanation of the origins of culture: of morality, of religion and of art. If we all have a sense of ourselves as helplessly disfigured in early childhood we must have a picture, a sense, of what it would be not to be so disfigured (the if-only life that will inform our grievance). Something was done to us – or, as in Richard's case, it was as though something was done to us – and we were helpless; either what was done couldn't be helped, or no help was available. Helpless means unprotected. It means, in this context, having an impotence foisted upon us, and organizing a life around this fact.

In this story it is clearly not part of our narcissism, part of our self-love, to be helpless in this way; or it is part of a negative narcissism, the specialness conferred by an exceptional suffering. And if it wasn't for this helplessness we would not suffer in the way we do. What is being conjured here is a counter-image of invulnerability, the opposite of helplessness. In this equation, it is our helplessness that makes us so narcissistically vulnerable, that makes our self-love so precarious. The nothing that can come from not being all. 'The hell of the narcissist is the tyranny of his need for others'; there is helplessness, in other words, but there is also the lure of self-sufficiency, of creating the illusion of being everything to oneself. And yet, of course, in a certain sense, helplessness is where we start from; or, as object relations theorists put it, dependence is where we start from. Either way we can't get round the fact that, as Winnicott put it, all philosophers were once babies. I want to consider in this essay Freud's story about helplessness with a view to making a case for it; that is, as a case for helplessness as something we shouldn't want to think of ourselves as growing out of. We can become more competent but we shouldn't imagine that we become less helpless. The wonderful phrase 'learned helplessness' reminds us, of course, that if helplessness can be learned, it can also be unlearned.

'Moral philosophy,' Charles Taylor wrote in *Sources of the Self*,

> has tended to focus on what it is right to do rather than on what it is good to be, on defining the content of obligation rather than the nature of the good life ... it has no conceptual place left for the notion of the good as the object of our love or our alle-

giance or, as Iris Murdoch portrayed it in her work, as 'the privileged focus of attention or will'.

In psychoanalysis the question, I think, has always been about what it is right to do about helplessness, rather than about helplessness as integral to the nature of the good life; or, indeed, as the object of our love or our allegiance. I think it should be the privileged focus of our attention, though probably not of our will. In the story I will be telling – and that Freud in some ways tells and in some ways doesn't – acknowledgement of dependence is no more of a solution to helplessness than the injunction to pull up your socks. And this is partly because helplessness is more often than not assumed to be a problem (what we are suffering from) rather than a pleasure (a strength or a virtue). It is not something, as it were, that we cultivate. We do not think of development as a project in which we want to become increasingly helpless, or one in which we elaborate and sophisticate our capacity for helplessness. But should we?

One of the moral questions ushered in by psychoanalysis is: what kind of good are the things we can't help but say, or do, or feel, or think, or desire? To which it is worth adding this further question: what good is helplessness? This is the question that perhaps inevitably exercised Freud; indeed virtually everything Freud wrote was not only about what can't be helped, and what can; but also, and more interestingly, about the moral consequences of our helplessness. So, what is called helplessness, and what good, if any, could it be?

In a section of Freud's early *Project for a Scientific Psychology* entitled 'The Experience of Satisfaction' he is trying to give an account, in neuronal terms, of how the infant, the rudimentary person, manages the stimulation of appetite. It is an interesting passage not least because it shows Freud using the language of science in a way that leads him into the language of morality; in the terminology of the *Project* we see that once the experience of satisfaction becomes the topic, the language of neurology becomes permeable to moral preoccupations; what Freud calls 'relief of tension' or 'discharge' turn inevitably into questions about the Good, about adequate ethical objects and 'moral motives'. Freud is working out an account, though this is not how he would have put it, of what the philosopher Alasdair MacIntyre calls 'the distinctive virtues of dependent rational animals, whose dependence, rationality and animality have to be understood in relationship to each other'. When Freud talks of the experience of satisfaction he is talking in the first instance of what is conducive to survival, and in the second instance, to put it rather more ambitiously, about what might be conducive to human flourishing. 'Satisfaction' is the word, the experience, that links what we have learned to call our desire and our obligation. And Freud, unsurprisingly, can't talk about any of this without invoking the idea of helplessness; without, indeed, making the helplessness of the human infant the heart of the matter. 'Experience shows,' Freud writes in *The Origins of Psychoanalysis*, keeping things as empirical as possible, that once appetite occurs:

> the first path to be followed is that leading to internal change (e.g., emotional expression, screaming, or vascular innervation). But ... no discharge of this kind can bring about any relief of tension, because endogenous stimuli continue to be received in spite of it ... Here a removal of the stimulus can be effected only by an intervention which will temporarily stop the release of quantity in the interior of the body, and an intervention of this kind requires an alteration in the external world (e.g., the supply of nourishment or the proximity of the sexual object), and this, as a 'specific action', can be brought about only in particular ways. At early stages the human organism is incapable of achieving this specific action. It is brought about by extraneous help, when the attention of an experienced person has been drawn to the child's condition by a discharge taking place along the path of internal change [e.g., by the child's screaming]. This path of discharge thus acquires an extremely important secondary function – viz., of bringing about an understanding with other people; and the original helplessness of

human beings is thus the primal source of all moral motives.

When the extraneous helper has carried out the specific action in the external world on behalf of the helpless subject, the latter is in a position, by means of reflex contrivances, immediately to perform what is necessary in the interior of his body in order to remove the endogenous stimuli. This total event then constitutes an 'experience of satisfaction', which has the most momentous consequences in the functional development of the individual.

The picture is of the desiring 'helpless subject' filling from within with the stimuli of hunger and seeking in the first instance relief through physical expression; this reflex magic fails because the stimuli of desire keep coming. What Freud calls 'the release of quantity' can be effected only by an intervention by someone else, someone outside. This 'specific action' – put in inverted commas by Freud – 'can be brought about only in particular ways': the supply of nourishment or the arrival of the sexual object, depending upon the attentiveness, the quality of attention from someone else, and their generosity. The essential thing, without which the child quite literally would not survive, is provided by someone else. Desire is made viable by its recipient. It is worth noting that by equating here, in this way, the supply of nourishment with the proximity of the sexual object, Freud is making them equally urgent needs; making us wonder what happens to the sexually desiring subject, the 'helpless subject', as Freud calls her, if her sexual need is not attended to, given that we know what happens to the unattended baby. But it is, in some ways, a simple point: the helpless subject needs help. Help is not something added on afterwards; it is integral. There is no position, no stage or state before helplessness; and there is no stage before what we call help is required. But then Freud makes his remarkable statement, almost as an afterthought: 'This path of discharge' – that is, the scream, the emotional expression – 'thus acquires an extremely important secondary function – viz., of bringing about an understanding with other people; and the original helplessness of human beings is thus the primal source of all moral motives.' The first function of the scream is an attempt at evacuation, at discharge of stimuli, which can't work; but the secondary function is as an appeal, a medium of communication or contact, between the 'helpless subject' and the person looking after her. It brings about an understanding with other people presumably because it stimulates the other person to work out, to imagine, what it might be that the helpless subject is in need of. It makes the other person think about what might be good for the helpless subject; and presumably about whether it would be good for them to try to provide what is needed.

'The original helplessness,' Freud writes, '... is thus the primal source of all moral motives.' 'Moral motives' might be construed as predispositions, or reasons, or causes to pursue the good. It is a usefully ambiguous phrase in the translation; is the original helplessness of human beings the primal source of all moral motives in the infant as helpless subject, or does the infant's helplessness – and the sexual adult's helplessness – call up moral motives in the recipient? Does our original helplessness make us moral, or is morality prompted in us by the way we respond to dependent others? It must be both. Freud is making a link between our original helplessness and the primal source of all moral motives; it is as though he is saying, without original helplessness there would be no moral motives. As though, however it works, morality is what we have invented, what has been summoned up in us, by our helplessness. Because we are originally helpless subjects – though by linking the hungry infant with the desiring sexual adult Freud is more than intimating not merely an original help-lessness, but an enduring or constitutive helplessness – we can't separate out obligation from need; we cannot help but consider what we need to do to, for and with the people upon whom we depend. To be a helpless desiring subject is to be implicated in, to be enmeshed in, and inextricable from, a world of moral considerations. And one of the things, of course, that this will involve us in are attempts – however forlorn or desperate or intermittent – to want to separate out desire and obligation. The way we tend to do this is to disavow helplessness. Once we keep helplessness in the picture – and put it, as Freud does, in the middle of the picture – we can't dissociate appetite and morality. You can say, as Richard does, 'I am myself alone' as a boast rather than as a statement of despair only if you have found a way of creating the illusion that you are not, in any way, what Freud calls a 'helpless subject', a subject who needs help; who is, indeed, only a subject at all because he has been helped. It is original helplessness that leads us to, that makes necessary, the idea of the Good.

But, of course, Freud doesn't say the original helplessness of human beings is thus the primal source of all *good* moral motives; he simply says morality is *bound up* with helplessness. It is worth recalling Charles Taylor's comment, quoted earlier, that 'Moral philosophy has tended to focus on what it is right to do rather than on what it is good to be, on defining the content of obligation rather than the nature of the good life.' Morality, we might say now, is what we have tended to do with original helplessness: morality is what we have made out of it. It is, at least in Freud's view – but these are my words not his – our self-cure, for better and for worse, for the fact that we are helpless subjects (and, Freud would add, helplessly sexual subjects). And the problem, we might say, is that we have tended to be – or have been

tempted or inclined to be, for reasons which we will
discuss – more like Richard; and by that I mean we
could begin to see that much of our discontent with
morality, much of our sense, when it exists, that morality is alien rather than integral, a foreign body foisted on
us to deprive us of our real satisfaction, comes from the
ways in which we can use morality to deny, abolish,
refuse, disparage, trivialize and punish our original
helplessness. Or to put it the other way round: any
morality that does not affirm, desire and value helplessness is merely punitive. That any morality that is not on
the side of helplessness – that can't bear to see its pleasures and its strengths – is going to feel estranging. So we
need to consider what might have to happen to original
helplessness that might make it a vice rather than a virtue, a persecution rather than a boon. What would make
us so averse to what is so original about us?

At least in the passage from the *Project*, Freud has a
fairly obvious answer to this question: helplessness
becomes persecution, is made into a problem, by being
insufficiently responded to. If the hungry infant's
needs are not at least recognized, if not always actually
met; if the sexually desiring adult finds no object
attentive to her desire, helplessness becomes intol-
erable; something has to be done with it (it might
be turned into omnipotence, say, or bitter, scornful,
mocking behaviour, which may be the same thing).
This is the reassuring, commonsensical account, one
that has been taken up in various versions of object

relations theory. It is not our nature that is the problem, but it is our parenting that can make it so.

You will notice in this account that helplessness is the precondition for being helped; as an experience in itself – as in the developmental theories of psychoanalysis – helplessness is not a good one; it is what it leads to that is of paramount importance – that is, the possibility of being understood and the generation, or evocation, of all moral motives. Helplessness is the precondition for human bonds, for exchange; you have to be a helpless subject in order to be helped, in order to be understood, in order to become a moral creature. And so, by the same token, if you can't experience helplessness you are precluded from these fundamental human experiences. To get back, or to be brought back, to helplessness is to be brought back to these things. So we shouldn't underestimate, from this point of view, the conscious or unconscious desire for helplessness that must exist alongside the wish to refuse it. We could, indeed, think of ourselves as suffering from an incapacity, or a refusal of states of helplessness, precisely because they reconnect us with these things that helplessness makes possible. (This is why states of illness can be so productive.) Logically, states of helplessness are to be avoided; Freud gives us a picture both of why they might be desired, and of the risks of desiring them. For Freud it is only this helpless subject that is capable of experiences of satisfaction, those experiences he describes as having

'momentous consequences in the functional development of the individual'. No helplessness, no satisfaction. Helplessness – which it is so difficult to find a
picture of for the adult that is not simply terrifying
– is the precondition for satisfaction. If we lose, or
forget, or repress, or project, or attack this original
helplessness, we quite literally lose, in Freud's terms,
the real possibilities for satisfaction. We become one
of the exceptions, like Richard.

Without helplessness there can be no possibility
of satisfaction, and without the possibility of satisfaction, there can be no aliveness, no point. Helplessness, Freud is suggesting, is the most important thing
about us. And yet, as he also says, helplessness is the
very thing we are prone to magic away, largely through
religion, but also through art and morality (and so, by
implication, by theory). If we can't bear helplessness
we can't bear satisfaction; there is a plot against helplessness, which turns out to be a plot against satisfaction. Real satisfaction, Freud implies, depends upon
living without illusions, without the wishful magic of
religious beliefs. The experience of satisfaction literally depends upon our living in Weber's disenchanted
world; a world without omnipotence in it. 'The
psychical origin of religious ideas,' Freud writes in
The Future of an Illusion:

... which are given out as teachings, are not precipi-
tates of experience or end results of thinking: they

are illusions, fulfilments of the oldest, strongest and most urgent wishes of mankind. The secret of their strength lies in the strength of those wishes. As we already know, the terrifying impression of helplessness in childhood aroused the need for protection – for protection through love – which was provided by the father; and the recognition that this helplessness lasts throughout life made it necessary to cling to the existence of a father, but this time a more powerful one. Thus the benevolent rule of a divine Providence allays our fears of the dangers of life; the establishment of a moral world-order ensures the fulfilment of the demands of justice, which have so often remained unfulfilled in human civilization; and the prolongation of earthly existence in a future life provides the local and temporal framework in which these wish-fulfilments shall take place.

This is, as many people have noticed, a rather sweeping account of religion. And though Freud is not saying, where religion was sex should be, he is wanting us to wonder what certain kinds of belief can do for us. But over thirty years after the *Project*, once again everything derives from the helplessness of childhood. But certain things have changed. First of all 'the original helplessness of human beings' has become, for the older Freud, 'the terrifying impression of helplessness in childhood'; and what this helplessness produces is not the experience of satisfaction, but the illusions of religion, with its all too plausible morality that is merely a wishful concealment of our real helplessness faced with the dangers of reality. Now helplessness only prompts us to obscure its existence; it is not the route to satisfaction but the root to a knowing self-deception. And this deception can be made complete only by wheeling on a spurious father figure. In the *Project* it was at least implied that the infant's helplessness would be met by the mother, and the adult's sexual desire would be met by a satisfying real object of no specified gender. Here, the solution to helplessness, which is in fact an evasion of it, is a faked-up father. Freud, we might infer, now believes that the majority of modern people can only turn against helplessness, satisfaction and truth; they take refuge in religion and its morality because – unlike that helpless subject of the *Project* – they can't bear, or bear with, their helplessness. It makes them invent a cartoon character, a parody, a man without disabilities, a man beyond help.

II

There is another world, but it is in this one.

Paul Éluard

There are, let us say, two solutions that Freud proposes to our original human helplessness: a good one and a bad one. In the good one, helplessness is the pre-condition for satisfaction – the only way to the experience of satisfaction; and by the same token the only way to morality. In the bad one, the experience of satisfaction is replaced by the experience of feeling protected. Helplessness issues in the wish to be protected from the experience of helplessness, not to feel it too acutely. Helplessness is not recognized, so to speak, as a predisposition towards sensuous satisfaction; it is as though someone has said, 'I need a drink,' and another person has replied, 'It's not a drink that you really need; you need your thirst to be made safe,' or as though someone has said, 'I'm hungry,' and the other person has replied, 'No, you're terrified.' So helplessness leads to satisfaction, or to self-deception; it produces understanding between people, or misunderstanding; and in both versions it leads to morality, the undisclosed morality of Freud's phrase in the *Project*, 'the primal source of all moral motives', or the morality Freud clearly despises, of the religiously consoled. It is, one might say, the difference between those who can bear being children and those who can't. Believing in religion is like believing that adulthood is the solution to childhood.

Religion, for Freud, is the false solution to human helplessness – the human helplessness that Freud is keen to insist lasts throughout life; it just begins in childhood – and satisfaction is the right solution, or perhaps we should say the right outcome (though sex, of course, is not going to solve all the problems religion addresses; for Freud, sexuality is anti-redemptive). But either way, all of what we think of as our moral problems spring from the fact that we are helpless subjects. And helplessness, or our relation to it, is something Freud thinks we need to get right; and we do the very worst things when we get it wrong; we start doing things like believing in God, or abiding by religious teachings, or adopting preposterous moralities. Or punishing/exploiting other people's vulnerabilities or ideologies, or believing that we are exceptional creations rather than just another species of animal. Obviously, if frustration makes us aggressive and we turn against our own satisfaction, we are unconsciously cultivating our violence by disavowing our helplessness.

Our fundamental response to our own helplessness is to create an enchanted world, a world of gods, a world in which we seek protection from our helplessness, but not engagement with it. 'Biologically speaking,' Freud writes in his paper on Leonardo Da Vinci,

> religiousness is to be traced to the small human child's long-drawn-out helplessness and need for help; and when at a later date he perceives how truly forlorn and weak he is when confronted with the great forces of life, he feels his condition as he did in childhood, and attempts to deny his own despondency by a regressive revival of the forces which protected his infancy.

It is almost as though the child underestimates her helplessness; or that what adulthood brings is a sense of just how helpless we really are. It is important, I think, that Freud nowhere suggests that we grow out of our helplessness – indeed, he suggests here that we grow *into* it – or that it is something that can be realistically overcome. For Freud, religion is a poor solution to an endemic, to a biological, problem; it is because we are helpless when confronted with what he calls 'the great forces of life' that we engage in this imaginative activity called religious belief. In Freud's view our helplessness doesn't diminish over time, but we become progressively more disturbed by it. So terrorized are we by it that we will seek safety rather than satisfaction, magic rather than nourishment, disavowal rather than acknowledgement. We seem, in Freud's view, to be the animals who are tormented by our helplessness; the animals for whom it is, or it has become, the abiding preoccupation. And in explaining this, in *Inhibitions, Symptoms and Anxiety*, Freud seems to allude to Richard III's soliloquy that he quoted in his paper on 'the exceptions'. 'The biological factor,' he writes, that makes us so prone to neuroses as a species,

> is the long period of time during which the young of the human species is in a condition of helplessness and dependence. Its intrauterine existence seems to be short in comparison with that of most animals,

and it is sent into the world in a less finished state. As a result, the influence of the real external world upon it is intensified and early differentiation between the ego and the id is promoted. Moreover, the dangers of the external world have a greater importance for it, so that the value of the object which alone can protect it against them and take the place of its former intrauterine life is enormously enhanced. The biological factor, then, establishes the earliest situations of danger and creates the need to be loved, which will accompany the child through the rest of its life.

Richard described himself as 'Deform'd, unfinish'd, sent before my time/ Into this breathing world'; Freud's human animal is too briefly in the womb, and 'sent into the world in a less finished state'. And Freud, of course, intimates that there may be a sense in which we are all deformed by our protracted helplessness and dependence. This left Richard with a grudge, and a supposed entitlement to avenge himself, at least in Freud's view. What is the grudge, what form does the revenge of the human animal take? The value of the object that can protect it is 'enormously enhanced', and the need to be loved will accompany the child through the rest of her life. What sense does it make to think of ourselves as deformed by our dependence? What picture of ourselves might we have if we were not so deformed, not suffering from what the poet Henri Cole calls the 'disease of imperfection'? The long period of time that the human species is 'in a condition of helplessness and dependence' leads to what we might call an idealization of the protecting object (that is, an unrealistic apprehension of it), and a cravenness, an enslavement to being loved (Richard we might think of as idealizing himself, and enslaved to being hated). This helplessness, which accompanies us through life, calls up in us the wish for a protective object that distorts perception, and a terror of loss of love. In other words, at its best, under one kind of description, our helplessness involves us with others, it weaves us into the human community; but at its worst, under another description, it makes us abject and infinitely exploitable creatures (we will do anything for love and protection). It is as though our original helplessness, the defining feature of ourselves throughout our lives, at worst corrupts us; and at best makes us morally pragmatic rather than moralistically principled. If we live in a condition of dependence and helplessness, and if what this leads us into is spurious, self-deceiving religious consolation, or the secular equivalents, how could we not end up hating our (and other people's) helplessness? How could we not end up thinking the absurd paradoxical thought, that the very thing that makes us what we are ruins our lives? This, at least, is one of the places that Freud leaves us. The catastrophe of being a human being is that we are irredeemably helpless creatures. And that means, helpless to do anything about our helplessness. We are essentially helpless, and that is the very thing that makes our lives impossible. It is a mark of our own resistance to our helplessness that we deem the ineluctable to be catastrophic; as though anything we don't make for ourselves is bad for us.

III

That innate incompetence, which Hooker ...
called 'this our imbecillitie'.

Geoffrey Hill, 'The Eloquence of Sober Truth'

Freud is making a distinction – though over time it is a distinction that gets lost – that at first sight seems rather crude: our original helplessness leads either at best to the experience of satisfaction, or at worst to the experience of religious belief, to essential sensual satisfactions of appetite, or to magic. But in making this distinction, by setting up these 'contraries' (to use Blake's term), Freud is opposing protection to satisfaction, not merely religion to sex. Our helplessness – that is, the helplessness of appetite – can lead us in the direction of the experience of satisfaction provided by attentive others; or our helplessness – our helplessness in the face of the dangers of the external world and the 'great forces of life', among which is appetite – can lead us in the direction of protection from unreal figures and magical beliefs. But this is not simply a version of our need for safety contending with our need for excitement. Freud is saying that our helplessness can force us into sacrificing – sacrificing by displacing – the experience of satisfaction; which, for Freud, in his early formulation in the *Project*, is itself a fundamental precondition for psychic and physical survival. The experience of helplessness, in other words, can make us sacrifice our lives, can lure us into a nihilistic pact: if you give up on the experience of satisfaction, you can be protected. Of course, we don't want it to be as stark as this; we can, as we say, have it both ways; and yet Freud, I think, is revealing a harsher truth: that there is something about our experience of helplessness – that there is, perhaps, something about the way helplessness is described, is presented in our culture, at this time – that makes us want to give up on our desire, and for something that can supposedly reassure us, but not fundamentally satisfy us. The quest for the experience of satisfaction may leave us unprotected; and we may give up on satisfaction in order not to face this reality.

So something about our helplessness, or its descriptions, may precipitate us into a delirium of compulsive protection-seeking; as though we believe we can be protected from the great forces of life. In Freud's view we are the animals who are uniquely vulnerable, oversensitive, one might say, to what living entails; we are sent into the world in a 'less finished state' than other animals, the dangers of the external world have a greater importance for us, and we require barriers between ourselves and our desire; as Freud puts it, 'early differentiation between the ego and the id is promoted'. Is this special pleading? In this account, are we, rather like Richard, the exceptions, but in this case the exceptions in the whole of nature? It is not, of course, difficult to see why Freud, at the time and place of writing, should feel his own and other people's unsuitedness or ill-fittingness to the world they found themselves in. Protection would be privileged over satisfaction for Jews and many others in Europe in the 1920s and 1930s; fundamental human satisfactions would feel increasingly remote. There would be what we might think of, in short, as new forms of helplessness, new pictures and experiences of helplessness – political, economic and, in Freud's language, psychic. And these very experiences could lead to radical redescriptions of the helplessness of infancy; of what the consequences of helplessness can be. Helplessness could only become horrifying; it might be increasingly difficult to find – and perhaps it has always been – inspiring pictures of helplessness, or accounts of helplessness that would make it sound, in Charles Taylor's words, something 'good to be', an object of our 'love' or our 'allegiance'.

No one says things now like, 'He's a wonderfully

helpless man,' or 'There was something impressively helpless about the way she dealt with that.' And yet Freud, I think, was beginning, in the *Project*, to make the case, or a case, for helplessness; for the fact that without the experience of helplessness there could be no possibility of the experience of satisfaction. Without the possibility of the experience of satisfaction, life is futile. Indeed, one way of seeing what Freud thinks of as the magic of religious belief is that it contains a long-term wish within it: that one day I will feel sufficiently protected so I will be able to get back to, to start up again, the quest for the experience of satisfaction. I will be able to sort out my helplessness – secure myself from it – so the life of appetite can begin again. But in the meantime I am going to have to believe in God. The fantasy of ultimate redemption, at least in psychoanalytic terms, might mean a disguised picture of when I can allow myself to start desiring again, in the belief my desire will be met, in the belief that there will be nothing self-destructive, nothing self-endangering, about my desire. In Freud's picture of appetite both sexual and other in the *Project*, to desire, to be hungry or sexually alive, is to risk one's life. An education in helplessness – if such a thing were possible; you might say we are always already overeducated in helplessness – would be an education in mortal risk.

Clearly a lot depends on what we feel about helplessness, on what, to put it as confoundingly as possible,

can be done about it, or with it. Could we, for
example, in the pragmatist way – which is not often
the psychoanalytic way – use it to get from A to B
without the very idea of using it becoming a denial
of its nature? What – to use William James's language
– might helplessness be good for? In the *Project*, after
all, Freud was telling us that helplessness was good
for the experience of satisfaction. That that is what it
was good for and that was what it was originally
meant for.

Of course, it seems odd to instrumentalize helplessness; but perhaps this is something we can't help
but do, and this, in itself, may be instructive. Freud
says, in the instances I have cited, that helplessness
is good for the experience of satisfaction, and good
for making us magical (that is, religious); it makes
us enchant the world with supernatural agents and
forces: amazingly powerful mothers and fathers, men
and women of our dreams. But Freud is also saying
that helplessness never stops; that in fact we get progressively more helpless. So we might say helplessness is only temporarily transformed by satisfaction,
but that religious belief creates the illusion that it is
permanently transformed (we are helpless, but our
helplessness is grounded by help, the infinite help of
God). Developmental theory fobs us off with the
sense that helplessness can be progressively transformed. Because what Freud is urging us to imagine
is what our lives would be like if we lived as if we

were all helpless all the time; and that this helplessness was the very thing we sought to conceal, or obscure, or deny; that our helplessness has no solution, there is no holding it at bay or growing out of it; that prior to sexuality or aggression or dependence there is helplessness as a way of life, a way of being. That we are helplessly desiring creatures. That our original (in both senses) and fundamental helplessness could be recognized, acknowledged, and even to some extent met – indeed, this is where object relations theory, attachment, relational psychoanalysis and other stories about dependence come in. But in all these pictures our helplessness is not temporarily relieved or assuaged or removed, it is just that so-called relationship is one of the things we do with, or about, our abiding and presiding helplessness. And if helpless is simply what we are – there is no other way of being, no way of being anything else – how and why have we made it such a problem? Or, to put it the other way round, why have we not seen it, in Taylor's words, as something 'good to be', not just bad to be? Indeed, we have, in a sense, defined the Good as that which relieves us of our helplessness, or makes it bearable, but without supposedly abolishing it. So when Charles Taylor asks, in *Sources of the Self*, 'What is it about the [human] subject that makes him recognize and love the good?' the answer could be: our helplessness makes the good, and the idea of the good, integral, indeed essential, to our survival and well-being – whether the good is God, or the mother, or ideological commitment, or moral conviction, or, as we say, the meeting of needs.

There is an obvious religious point here, which has broader implications. 'Fallen man was utterly helpless,' Taylor writes, 'and could do nothing by himself. The point of harping on the helplessness and depravity of mankind was to throw into the starkest relief the power and mercy of God, who could bring about a salvation which was utterly beyond human power and, what is more, still wanted to rescue his unworthy creature beyond all considerations of justice.' Our helplessness then, in this usefully generalizable description – for God, here, we could put the mother, the parental couple, the saving ideology, and so on – is the precondition for our idea of the good; one could almost say it makes the idea of the good possible, even plausible. Without our original helplessness such a thing would never have occurred to us. But there is a familiar moral move here that is worth noting: helplessness has to be characterized as 'depravity' (to use Taylor's term), or lack, or weakness, to make the good look good. It is reminiscent of Nietzsche's striking point in *On the Genealogy of Morals* when he writes of our 'will to establish an ideal – that of the "holy God" – and to feel the palpable certainty of [our] unworthiness with respect to that ideal'. What if our casting of helplessness as weakness, as a form of depravity, has produced spurious forms of strength, of the good as that which relieves us of, or even conceals, our helplessness? When Freud implies in the *Project* that we can satisfy each other but not save each other, we might take him to be saying: satisfaction, cumulatively experienced – or even satisfaction risked – can make helplessness a strength. Indeed, if, as Freud does, you make the experience of satisfaction, and the frustration that leads to it, into the constitutive human experiences, then helplessness – that is, the helplessness of appetite, of desiring – is our fundamental strength. Without it there is no frustration and no possibility of the experience of satisfaction. Is helplessness only a good if and when we are helped?

So, if the Good was to be formulated not as an overcoming of helplessness, or a compensation for it, or a denial of it; if the Good, in other words, was not itself believed to be without helplessness (as God is), what would it be like? And my invoking of Nietzsche's *Genealogy of Morals* is, of course, a warning in the background, because the risk is, in promoting helplessness as a virtue, as an original strength, that we might simply be elaborating what Nietzsche calls, in his distasteful and exhilarating way, the 'slave revolt in morals', the tyranny of the weak over the strong, what he thinks of as the corrupt and corrupting 'intelligence introduced by the powerless'. Can we, in his terms, 'approach the problems of morality in high spirits' by making the case for helplessness, or does considering the sheer scale of our helplessness make us feel weaker; as though even talking about helplessness could drive us to despair, or to sentimentality, or to object relations, or to drink? Why, in short, does helplessness make us think of consolation rather than inspiration? Why is it associated in our minds more with being tortured than being high-spirited, with being desperate rather than being available, with sadomasochism rather than with abandon?

'You can either resent the way life is ordained, or be intrigued by it,' wrote the critic Denis Donoghue. I think we are inclined – and perhaps even encouraged, even educated – to resent our helplessness, to be frightened of it rather than intrigued by it. There is, of course, one sense in which our helplessness is not ordained: we are not born helpless, we become helpless. For the first years of our life it never occurs to us that helpless is what we are. Helplessness is something that, over time, we learn about ourselves; it becomes the word we might use for certain experiences. And then, it seems, once we have got the idea, helplessness becomes the thing, the condition, that we are always trying to do something about. Because we seek to relieve our helplessness we think of it as something that we suffer, or suffer from. But what if we thought of ourselves as getting progressively more helpless as we got older? And of helplessness as something we grow into, partly by becoming aware of it? In order to do this we might have to broaden the analogy horizon. After all, we don't think of ourselves as relieving our need for oxygen by breathing, whereas we do think of ourselves as relieving our hunger with food. We can't satisfy our need not to be helpless.

So, by way of conclusion I have two suggestions, both I hope in the spirit of Freud's 'The Creative Writer and Daydreaming'. 'The true ars poetica,' Freud writes in this paper, 'lies in the technique by which [the artist] overcomes our repulsion, which certainly has to do with the barriers that arise between each single ego and the others.' I take it that there is something about our helplessness – the pictures we have of ourselves as helpless – that we find repulsive; and that the barriers that arise between each single ego and the others is, in part at least, a consequence of our disavowal of our original helplessness, which is the thing we have most originally in common with each other, such that the acknowledgement of this helplessness in common makes all such barriers between us seem wildly unrealistic. My two suggestions are first: that any psychoanalysis that privileges knowing over being, insight over experience, narrative over incoherence, diminishes if not actually forecloses our real acknowledgement of helplessness. If we could think of our helplessness as like a figure inside us – as, to use Hilary Putnam's phrase from another context, 'a being who breaks my categories' – we could not only be trying to overcome it but, as Freud intimates in the *Project*, we could also be trying to sustain it. We could think of our helplessness as sustaining us. There being nothing else, ultimately, that could do so. It would not simply be one of the best things about us, but it would be *the* thing, the condition without which we could not be who we are. In this picture, there is no version of ourselves that is not helpless, even if, in different areas of our lives, there are different forms of helplessness, and we are helpless in different ways. We can be competent but we are always helpless.

My second suggestion, following on from this, is that helplessness leads us too automatically into talking about dependence (and now, of course, attachment). When I was working on a ward for children with cancer a mother once said to me, pointing to her daughter asleep in a hospital bed, 'We are relying on her now.' After all the doctors, after all the help that is available, we are ultimately helplessly dependent on our own bodies, on their sustaining vitality or lack of it. No other body is available but the body we happen to be. There can be virtues in necessity. And in the fact that there are necessities.

III The Perfectionist

O great and wonderful happiness of man! It is given
to him to have that which he desires, and to be that
which he wills.

Giovanni Pico della Mirandola,
Oration on the Dignity of Man (1486)

They are called perfectionists, and this is often how
they describe themselves. And it is never clear
whether this is a boast ('my standards are so high and
my talents so extraordinary') or a kind of regret ('my
life is tyrannized by this neurotic obsession'). Either
way, and it is usually both, depending on the person's
mood, there is some demand that has to be met, some
rules, however obscure, to be followed; scruples or
principles that cannot be set aside. As a patient the
perfectionist – whether he is an artist or a bureaucrat,
a lawyer or a chemist – is never merely an obsessional
person. No one knows better than the perfectionist
the resistances in his chosen medium, the way it can
baffle his desire, and liberate it beyond his wildest
dreams. No one knows more than the perfectionist
about his own abjection, his own unrelenting incapacity to be as good as he should be. And so the perfectionist often assumes – like his counterpart, the

so-called pervert – that to be cured of his symptom
would be to lose his life; his disdain for the people
who care rather less – for the parts of himself that
have dispensed with this tyrannical ambition – is
often chilling. The Perfectibility of Man, that great
Renaissance and Enlightenment project, may be
everywhere ironized today, but the perfectionists are
still with us, with their ambivalent complaint. For the
perfectionist, to be 'good enough' is to be no good.
For the perfectionist, for example, there could be no
such thing as a good-enough mother.

What the perfectionist knows about, what the perfectionist is trying to ward off as both knowledge and
experience is, in Winnicott's language, catastrophic
disillusionment (the nothing that comes from not
being all). The perfectionist knows that there is incapacity, insufficiency, incompetence – but it must not
be in him. Or, rather, because it is in him all the time
– whose potential for self-hatred is greater than the
perfectionist's? – he must work against it. Just as most
mothers know that there is no such thing as the perfect mother, but most mothers want to be much more
than good enough; similarly, all perfectionists realize
that perfection is not possible. They are the victims
par excellence of an unrealistically intractable ego-
ideal; and they are knowingly the victims of this
impossible project, which is part of their torment (for
these people it is a rationalization to say that it is better
to travel hopefully than to arrive). Their incapacity is,

by definition, the problem; that it could be a solution to anything – or even a kind of strength or resource – is virtually unimaginable.

Our gods are never resourceless. 'What is God?' the catechism asks: 'God is the Supreme Spirit, Who alone exists of Himself, and is infinite in all perfections.' To be perfect, whatever else it is, is to be like God, of boundless perfection (God is not someone in search of self-improvement). The perfectionist is always an ever-failing god, never merely a struggling animal. Given that omnipotence is an all-or-nothing affair – you can no more be a bit omnipotent than you can be a bit pregnant – there is going to be no one more enraged than a failing god. And the theme of the failed god – whether it is Milton's Satan, or Goethe's Mephistopheles – is insufficiency; either its denial, or its presence felt through envy and retaliation. Helplessness is an experience that is available only to those who were once omnipotent; lack is an experience that is available only to those who were once, if only in fantasy, complete. From a psychoanalytic point of view it is the wound of need that constitutes the human subject. And Freud's question was: how has it come about that the human subject experiences his need as a wound, his desire as an insufficiency? Why is insufficiency an insult to the ego, rather than its greatest virtue? What psychoanalysis adds to the conversation is the idea that the wish for perfection is a derivative of the wish for self-sufficiency.

There is, Freud intimates in *Beyond the Pleasure Principle*, something enigmatic about how bewitched we are by the idea of perfection. If it doesn't represent merely the overcoming of all suffering, or the ultimate narcissistic refuge, what might it capture, what might it represent for us, this prevailing wish to be, as it were, so much better than we are? Or, rather, to be something other than we are, creatures with limited resources, creatures of scarcity? What is the ambition, the drive to be perfect, an ambition for? This is Freud's implicit question. Perfectionism must be of extraordinary significance given how difficult, historically, it has been to renounce (it is impossible to imagine a person not in the grip, in some way, of the fantasy of perfection). 'It may be difficult,' Freud writes with a certain understatement,

> for many of us to abandon the belief that there is an instinct towards perfection at work in human beings, which has brought them to their present high level of intellectual achievement and ethical sublimation and which may be expected to watch over their development into supermen. I have no faith, however, in the existence of any such internal instinct and I cannot see how this benevolent illusion is to be preserved. The present development of human beings requires, as it seems to me, no different explanation from that of animals. What appears in a minority of individuals as an untiring impulsion towards further perfection

can easily be understood as a result of the instinctual repression upon which is based all that is most precious in human civilization. The repressed instinct never ceases to strive for complete satisfaction, which would consist in the repetition of a primary experience. No substitutive or reactive formations and no sublimations will suffice to remove the repressed instinct's persisting tension; and it is the difference in amount between the pleasure of satisfaction which is demanded and that which is actually achieved that provides the driving factor which will permit of no halting at any position attained ...

That there could be an 'instinct towards perfection' is a way of marking rhetorically the power of the progress myth that Freud wants to unsettle. This 'benevolent illusion', in his view, has been integral to the project of uprooting the human from its animality; once it is acknowledged that we are not like animals but that we *are* animals the explanation of this 'untiring impulsion towards future perfection' becomes clear. Perfection is when the satisfaction demanded by the instinct is achieved; perfection is when there is no gap between desire and consummation. Perfection in the cultural sphere – or in so-called personal life – is a displacement of the wish for the repetition of 'a primary experience' of satisfaction. Freud makes it quite clear that no substitution, no reaction formation, no sublimations, can diminish or appease the instinct's tension, its persistent drive towards satisfaction. The fantasy of perfection, in other words, is the imaginative elaboration of a primary experience of satisfaction (or of wished-for satisfaction). The wish for perfection is an unconscious acknowledgement of the impossibility of repeating primary experiences of satisfaction. Or an acknowledgement that they did not exist, that satisfaction is always lacking.

Kleinians might want to say that perfectionism is a failed, a distracted, form of mourning; that what is there to be mourned, so to speak, is infantile omnipotence, the saboteur, in the Kleinian schema, of development. But what Freud is saying is that this is something we can't mourn, or learn to accept, or even fully acknowledge; this wish to repeat the primary experience of satisfaction, and the impossibility of this repetition, even when it is known about – it cannot be known but only known about – is our fundamental experience of ourselves. This discrepancy, this incongruity between demand and achievement, is something, at least in Freud's view, we must live with. There are no substitutions, no reaction formations, no sublimations, he insists, that could possibly work. 'The backward path,' he writes ruefully, 'that leads to complete satisfaction is as a rule obstructed by the resistances that maintain the repressions.' There is no complete satisfaction and only complete satisfaction is wanted. The only problem with desire is that it involves frustration; and frustration, whatever else it is, is an acknowledgement of incapacity. It is, Freud suggests, a capacity for incapacity that is required. Incomplete satisfaction is our fate but there are individuals for whom the only project is complete satisfaction; not 'every human being', Freud asserts, has this 'instinct towards perfection', and he quotes, by way of illustration, Mephistopheles in Goethe's *Faust*, who 'Presses forward ever unsubdued', speaking up for the daemonic power of this instinct towards perfection, this demand for complete satisfaction.

Are perfectionists then the people who have never given up on desire? Or are they realists, the unconscious ironists of their own desire; that is, of its impossibility? Perhaps, in the service of development as object relations theory would suggest, the idea of complete satisfaction should be mourned, or simply, more realistically, replaced by the idea of good-enough satisfaction? What we never lose, Freud insists, is the wish for complete satisfaction. It is not desiring per se that is the problem, it is being able to bear, and bear with, the inevitable repetition of incomplete satisfaction.

There is, then, the impossibility of recovering the supposed satisfaction of what Freud calls the 'primary experience', and the untiring wish to do so; and there is the Oedipus complex, which is linked in with this formative impossibility. Frustration, in other words, is our primary preoccupation, our 'essential perplexity' (to use Borges's phrase from a different context). We must ask not simply the essentially pragmatic questions: what can we do with our frustration? What can we make of it (or with it)? What, if anything, can we transform it into or use it to do? But also, what makes us phobic of frustration? – a question that cannot be answered by simply saying that frustration always portends an excess of frustration, or calls up the very feelings we cannot bear (rage, envy, spite, abjection, and so on). If psychoanalysis insists that the incapacity to bear frustration sabotages the individual's development, it needs, by the same token, to make the case for resourcelessness – and if for no other reason than the fact that most so-called pathology, at least from a psychoanalytic point of view, can be summed up as false solutions, or, rather, poor solutions, to resourcelessness, to a fundamental intolerance of incapacity. What we call pathologies are often self-cures for frustration. The most difficult thing for the patient to articulate is the nature of his frustration; indeed, he can only begin to articulate his desire if he can spell out his frustration. The idealizing in contemporary culture – and not only in contemporary culture – of the resourceful individual, of the person who knows what he wants and how to get it, is an acknowledgement of this now widespread terror of frustration.

Freud, in what looks now like an unusually prescient paper, 'Those Wrecked by Success' (the second section of his article 'Some Character-Types Met with in Psychoanalytic Work'), begins by suggesting the obvious: 'Psychoanalytic work has furnished us with the thesis that people fall ill of a neurosis as a result of frustration.' Illness is caused by dissatisfaction, as though in protest, as though frustration was against the natural order. And yet, Freud goes on to say, 'people occasionally fall ill precisely when a deeply rooted and long-cherished wish has come to fulfilment'. For these people, or for these people with these particular wishes, frustration is a precondition of health. What 'psychoanalytic work teaches us', he concludes, 'is that the forces of conscience which induce illness in consequence of success, instead of, as normally, in consequence of frustration, are closely connected with the Oedipus complex, the relation to father and mother'. Frustration, unsuccess, incapacity are, in the light of the Oedipus complex – as heirs of the Oedipus complex, so to speak – the preconditions for health; it is about how to fail (or 'fail better', in Beckett's words). There is nothing more unrealistic than the wish to succeed, at least for 'these people'.

IV The Lost

We have to be as subtle as our memories. That's all.

Mary Butts, *Armed with Madness*

A total of close to ninety million people were
either killed or displaced in Europe between
the years 1939 and 1948.

Mark Mazower, *Dark Continent*

In some passages written in 1939 in preparation for
his study of Baudelaire, entitled 'Central Park', Walter Benjamin wrote: 'The labyrinth is the habitat of
the dawdler. The path followed by someone reluctant to reach his goal easily becomes labyrinthine. A
drive, in the stages leading to its satisfaction, acts
likewise. But so, too, does a humanity (a class) which
does not want to know where its destiny is taking
it.' The Labyrinth, traditionally, indeed mythically,
something built to get lost in – in which the lost
object is the exit, in which every destination depends
upon the way out – is, as Benjamin suggests, the
'habitat', the environment created by the person
who seeks to fustrate themselves. The way Benjamin

pictures this is that the dawdler, like the drive itself, because it knows what it wants, is reluctant to, as he says, reach its goal. Getting lost is what you do – is what the dawdler does – when he is in no way lost; when he knows exactly where he is going, and how to get there. Getting lost, the creation of the labyrinth, is the work done when there is an object of desire. You get lost because you are not lost. So we can say: we are lost when there is no object of desire; and we make ourselves lost when there is an object of desire. We get lost. It is something we get.

Of course, Benjamin, comparing a drive with the dawdler – 'a drive, in the stages leading to its satisfaction, acts likewise', that is, enters the labyrinth it makes – brings psychoanalysis into the picture, by association as it were. In Freud's work, the incest taboo is the name he gives to the fact that the child always knows where he is going, and has to do something about this. There is a sense in which, in Freud's account, the child is never lost because the child always knows where he wants to be and should be (they are the same). He can get lost on the way, but he knows where he is going. The Oedipus complex structures the child's desire – the directions in which he is drawn, the spaces he prefers – such that he can lose the object of desire but can't, in the ordinary course of things, lose his desire for it. The parents are loved and hated but they are always wanted. There is no place like home, not even home itself, because, at least to begin with, and always, there are no people like one's parents; or no people about whom one has the same feelings as one does about one's parents (and siblings). Everyone, let's say, has a thing about their mother. And a thing about their father. Because of the incest taboo the child knows where she is going but mustn't get there; and the adult doesn't know where it is going and must get there. So the so-called resolution of the Oedipus complex, insofar as such a thing is possible – the relinquishing, the abjuring, of one's desire for the parents, without the defeat or the betrayal of one's own desire – involves the freedom to be lost, rather than the need to make oneself lost. Because the child knows what he wants, he has to get lost; because the adult doesn't know what he wants, he is lost. Because the making of labyrinths is second nature, it is very difficult not to make them. Somebody dawdling in a labyrinth is a perfect image, as though this person has forgotten what he is doing there; as though for him, at least, this is no longer a labyrinth but a pleasant place to be walking. The means have become an end in themselves. It's not that travelling hopefully is better than arriving, but that travelling is there to protect you from the possibility of arrival. And psychoanalysis is effectively a dictionary of all the ways in which we travel to keep arrival at bay; of which getting lost is some kind of emblem. Benjamin's dawdler is like Lacan's obsessional neurotic: 'What in its various advances and many byways

the behaviour of the obsessional reveals and signifies,'
he writes in *The Ethics of Psychoanalysis*:

> is that he regulates his behaviour so as to avoid what he
> often sees quite clearly as the goal and end of his desire.
> The motivation of this avoidance is often extraordin-
> arily radical, since the pleasure principle is presented
> to us as possessing a mode of operation which is pre-
> cisely to avoid excess, too much pleasure.

For the obsessional, Lacan continues, 'the object
with relation to which the fundamental experience,
the experience of pleasure, is organized, is an object
which literally gives too much pleasure'. There are
two things here we should note; one obvious, one
less so: the obvious point is that the individual 'organ-
izes' himself 'fundamentally' around the experience
of pleasure and the object who provides it, or with
whom such pleasure is possible. Space, time and direction, in other words, are organized around this object
of desire; we are, in a simple sense, orientated by this
object of desire; we might imagine it as a tropism, an
affinity, a magnetic attraction and repulsion. This
object of desire is like the obstacle we can't get round;
we may be at a loss to hold its attention, or sustain its
desire, we may actually lose it, but it is always where
we want to go, even in our avoidance of it. Finding an
object of desire is like being discovered; like being
exposed. But once there is an object of desire the

individual is no longer lost, in this one sense; like the dawdler, or the obsessional, they know where they want to go even if they then devote their lives to not going there. The only problem the desiring individual has is how to get there.

And yet, of course – and this is the second, less obvious, point – once there is an object of desire there is a fantasy of catastrophe. Lacan says that for the obsessional the catastrophe is an excess of pleasure, for the hysteric an excess of frustration; in other words, once there is an object of desire there is an omniscient fantasy about the consequences of pursuing the object of desire. Those people Lacan calls obsessionals and hysterics live as if they know exactly what is going to happen if they achieve their goal; the future will replicate the past. Experience of the past becomes certainty about the future. The omniscient, needless to say, never feel lost; or, rather, the omniscient part of ourselves always knows what is happening and what is going to happen. The omniscient part of ourselves always knows where we are. Whether or not Lacan is right in his classification – and, of course, the rhetorical authority of his own categories is one form omniscience takes – it does seem to me to be useful, when talking about losing and getting lost, to talk about excess. That getting lost is an attempt to regulate some kind of excess, probably a different kind of excess for each person, but somewhere ranged along the pleasure–pain continuum.

So, by way of some opening propositions: children can, of course, get lost, but they always know where they want to be; because there is an incest taboo they have to realize something very difficult, which is that they know where they want to go, but they must not go there; they have to discover, they have to invent, the experience of getting lost. Adults, because there is no place like home – because there is an incest taboo they have to some extent given up the parents as objects of desire – are lost; adulthood is exchanging, and knowing the difference between, getting lost and being lost; between the artefact you must make, and the experience you are powerless to avoid. Children get lost, adults have the possibility of being lost; though they, we, will spend as much time as we can getting lost to protect ourselves from the experience of being lost. There is only one mother and father, but there are an unknowable number of objects of desire outside the family (we may grow up in a xenophobic nation state, but we grow up into a multiculture of other people).

Getting lost, I want to suggest, is our best defence against being lost; and partly because it makes us feel that we have, as it were, taken the problem into our own hands, turned, as psychoanalysts say, passive into active. We may idealize getting lost as a great adventure; we may create habitations that get us lost, or that, like labyrinths, we can lose ourselves in. But to put it as briefly as possible, we get lost when we are lost in a way we can't bear. We are lost when there is no object of desire, and we get lost when there is one. So being lost involves acknowledging the inevitable frustration of there being no one (or nothing) around that one wants, perceiving that traumatic reality; and getting lost might involve working out, as far as one can, what kind of excess not being lost supposedly involves one in. One gets lost when there is the excess of an object of desire in the vicinity; one is lost in the absence of this promising excess. So, to go a bit further, we need to ask what maps are for, maps that by definition are not the ground; and that means, among other things, that they are not excessive in the way the ground is. If they were, the map would be the ground.

There is a poem by the Czech poet and immunologist Miroslav Holub, in his 1984 collection, *On the Contrary and Other Poems*, entitled 'Brief Reflection on Maps':

Albert Szent-Gyorgi, who knew a thing or
    two about maps,
By which life moves somewhere or other,
Used to tell this story from the war,
Through which history moves somewhere or other:

From a small Hungarian unit in the Alps a young
    lieutenant
Sent out a scouting party into the icy wastes.

At once
It began to snow, it snowed for two days and the party
Did not return. The lieutenant was in distress: he
   had sent
His men to their deaths.

On the third day, however, the scouting party
   was back.
Where had they been? How had they managed to find
   their way?
Yes, the man explained, we certainly thought we were
Lost and awaited our end. When suddenly one of
   our lot
Found a map in his pocket. We felt reassured.
We made a bivouac, waited for the snow to stop, and
   then with the map
Found the right direction.
And here we are.

The lieutenant asked to see that remarkable map in
   order to
Study it. It wasn't a map of the Alps
But the Pyrenees.

Goodbye.

   Perhaps the most obviously puzzling things about
this wonderfully lucid parabolic poem are the first

words and the last, the beginning of the journey
and the end; the poem begins with a name, Albert
Szent-Gyorgi, and ends with the word 'Goodbye'.
Albert Szent-Gyorgi, for those of us who don't know
– and who therefore begin the poem a bit lost – won
the Nobel Prize for Physiology and Medicine in 1937.
If you Google him you discover the life of a remarkable man who made significant contributions to
research into cancer, muscle physiology, cell respir-
ation and vitamin C. He was also, in a way more evi-
dently pertinent to the poem, actively anti-Nazi in
Hungary, his country of origin, during the Second
World War, having fought in the First World War;
he had received the Silver Medal for Valour and was
discharged after being wounded in action in 1917. He
subsequently emigrated to America. So the sense in
which, as the poem says, 'Albert Szent-Gyorgi ...
knew a thing or two about maps,/ By which life
moves somewhere or other,' conflates the maps made
of the inside of the body in its struggle for survival,
and the maps required in wartime. Sentences and dia-
grams about the inner workings of the body are like
maps; and yet, the poem tells us, when these men got
lost what they needed was a map, possibly any map, a
map of anywhere. The map that rescued them in the
Alps was a map of the Pyrenees; maps can work, at
least if we are desperate enough, just by being maps.
They were 'lost' and awaited their 'end' until they
found a map; not *the* map.

What does the success story in this poem tell us maps are? Clearly we couldn't trust someone who said to us, all you need for this journey is a map, any map, or indeed a doctor who believed that you could treat a heart condition by learning about the liver. One thing the poem tells us is that what these desperate, lost men needed was a map; and, to extend this for my purposes here, we might say that in that predicament a map was the object of desire, and that, by the same token, an object of desire is a map. It gives you direction without your necessarily noticing what or who it is. They didn't need the map of where they were, the real map, to get back; they just needed one that gave them a sense of direction. As long as you have got a map, any map, you are no longer lost; as long as you have a certain kind of object of desire, you are no longer lost. We need a person to long for, an object of longing, because it orientates the excess, the complexity of our hearts and minds. If we were to reverse the ostensive meaning of the poem we might say being lost makes people unusually inventive in the use of their objects. These men could turn a map of the Pyrenees into a map of the Alps. Being lost made them so unrealistic that they survived; their frustration, their desperation, made them magicians, or perhaps alchemists.

Making the last line and the last word of a poem about people being lost the single word 'Goodbye' makes the word itself enigmatic. What, for example, does the word 'goodbye' have to do with maps, in this brief reflection on maps? There are, as there are supposed to be, several possibilities; but the one I want to entertain here is one that the structure of the poem suggests; this poem about getting lost, finding the wrong map and being found leads up to a goodbye. There is, we see, no commentary, no reflection on the stark truth that is discovered by the lieutenant; he 'asked to see that remarkable map in order to/ study it. It wasn't a map of the Alps/ But the Pyrenees.// Goodbye.' Goodbye, as if to say, this speaks for itself; or, goodbye to reality, or empirical reality. The lieutenant thought he had said goodbye to his men, and then discovered that because they could say goodbye to reality they were saved. An object of desire is a map, not the ground. And being lost is a state of excessive desire, desire so strong that it can distort reality in the service of psychical survival. If there is no object of desire around one has to be invented; the remarkable map has to be used as something that it is, a map, but recreated into something it isn't – a map of the Alps.

In this poem we assume that the men were not dawdling, they were not unconsciously getting lost, they were really lost. But in this instance the men are more like the child I described earlier, the one who knows where he wants to go; even if all objects of desire, all aims and directions, even survival itself, are tainted with the forbidden and are therefore in some way to be avoided, we take it that these men were doing the opposite; they were so keen to get back they made a map of the Pyrenees a map of the Alps. If getting lost is an avoidance of the object of desire, being lost may be the precondition for finding the object of desire. Getting to the pitch of frustration in which you make what you need. And clearly, though not coyly, Holub's 'Brief Reflection on Maps' is also a Brief Reflection on Writing Poems as well as a Brief Reflection on being Lost. The map will work only if we don't read it too closely, if we don't see what it really is. Being lost can make us usefully deluded, inventively careless, happily inattentive. So the poem makes us wonder what it is not to be lost, or what the experience of being lost is like such that it can make us successfully use a map of the Pyrenees as a map of the Alps. These are the falsifications that survival can require of us. The object of desire is a map we use according to our needs. It gives us a sense of direction at the cost of a sense of reality. Maps, according to the poem, give us a sense of direction by not telling us where we are. If they had seen that it was a map of the Pyrenees they would have been truly lost. You never know which goodbye will be the last one.

In Holub's poem the 'remarkable map' helps them once they are lost; but further reflection on maps reminds us that they are there to prevent us from getting lost; we use them to prepare for the getting lost that might occur. They tell us by showing us where we want to go; or, rather, we use the map either to find out how we get to where we want to go, or to find out where we may go. Like Holub's desperate men we are 'reassured' by them, if not insured, supposedly, against getting lost. Freud, for whom, perhaps interestingly, maps were not the thing – there are only seven references to them in his work – used them once as an interesting analogy, once again connected to war, and to the dangers of desire, of locating the object of desire. He is writing about how anxiety, as he puts it, 'makes repression', in the *New Introductory Lectures* of 1933. The question, as always for Freud, is of how the individual pursues his satisfaction without too much harm, without excessive loss. 'The ego,' he writes,

> notices that the satisfaction of an emerging instinctual demand would conjure up one of the well-remembered situations of danger. This instinctual cathexis must therefore be somehow suppressed, stopped, made powerless. We know that the ego succeeds in this task if it is strong and has drawn the instinctual impulse concerned into its organization. But what happens in the case of repression is that the instinctual impulse still belongs to the id and that the ego feels weak. The ego thereupon helps itself with a technique which is at bottom identical with normal thinking. Thinking is an experimental action carried out with small amounts of energy, in the same way

that a general shifts small figures about on a map
before setting his large body of troops in motion.

This 'experimental action' in thought is the way,
Freud writes, that 'the ego anticipates the satisfaction
of the questionable instinctual impulse and permits it
to bring about the reproduction of the unpleasurable
feelings at the beginning of the feared situation of
danger'. Thinking of the quest for satisfaction is a
rehearsal; as though one might gain power over the
fear by going on imagining the scene. And yet the
effect of the analogy of the general with his toy sol-
diers and map suggests just how forlorn, how naive,
the ego is compelled to be. The general can't not
use the map and small figures to prepare his strategy,
but the difference between the game and the reality is
stark. And in the game that the general plays before
the battle, the game that he cannot help but play, there
is one thing he is wanting to have some sway over;
and that is, the loss, in both senses, of his troops. The
map, as in the Holub poem, is a protective device; the
ego is in mortal danger from the instinctual impulse,
from the desire, and the map is slightly fobbing him
off, or tempting him, as if to say, if you look at it like
this, if we rehearse, if we go over it, it's not quite so
dangerous. The one thing that Freud knew about
war – in 1933 as we do now – is that it is inherently
unpredictable; as Holub remarks at the beginning of
his poem, it is 'war,/ Through which history moves

somewhere or other', that is, in an unknowable direction. Faced with that history-maker, a dangerous instinctual impulse – mortally dangerous in that its attempted satisfaction might involve castration or other terminal losses – the ego says to itself: what you need is a map, you need to practise (as though practise makes perfect). The map, as Holub's poem suggests in its own riddling way, is our best self-cure for loss. A map, even any map, protects us from losing and being lost. But as always the proposed solution tells us more about the problem than about its hoped-for resolution. The map tells us that we are already lost; we have maps in the first place because we don't know where we are, we don't know where there is to get to, and we don't know how to get there. Or, to make the problem rather more domestic, more familiar: if we have been lucky enough to escape the catastrophes of history we do not need a map to find our parents. Or at least we have survived because at the beginning we could get to our parents (or caretakers) and we knew that they were our necessary destination. In this sense, only children have homes; and an adult who feels at home in the world is out of touch with reality. Growing up means needing a map. Children shouldn't feel lost; adults should feel lost because that is what they are.

The battle that Freud's rather poignant general is preparing for is the battle of life in which dangerous instincts – instincts that are both transgressive and

that can lose us love – are contending with an antag-
onistic reality; what Stanley Cavell calls, 'Freud's
vision of the human animal's compromise with existence.' Freud's human animal's problem is that he is
not lost, in the sense that he knows what he wants
initially, the parents, the objects of incestuous desire;
but he is at a loss because he cannot have them. To
begin with, Freud's animal knew what he wanted and
therefore knew where he was going, then he realized
he couldn't go there; he realized that he had to go
somewhere else for something he could never get. To
make it formulaic: the Freudian animal begins not
being lost, is then at a loss, and is then lost. He begins
without a map because to all intents and purposes he
knows where he is and knows where he is going; then
eventually he needs a map because he no longer knows
where he is or where he is going. There is no place
like home, and if you don't go home where do you
go? Maps become a necessity, but they are frail, minimal things compared with the uncontrolled excesses
they depict. And so are objects of desire. Faced with
the object of desire and the feeling stirred we will
dawdle, we will make labyrinths and wander round
them happily, we will consult maps which are hand-
me-downs, or make our own maps. And these are all,
whatever else they are, reminders that we are losing
and getting lost.

Of course, the story I am telling about the Oedipus complex and its fate for the individual is never

as stark or as simple as: we begin knowing what
we want, then we know we mustn't have it, then we
renounce it, then we find something else instead. It is,
though, as stark as: there are only two parents but
there are, as I have said, an unknowable number of
other objects of desire outside the family. Growing
up does complicate our desire beyond our compre-
hension; childhood is the easiest period of our lives to
understand, if it is the life of desire that we want to
understand. 'The Oedipus complex,' Laplanche and
Pontalis write in their great dictionary, *The Language
of Psychoanalysis*, 'plays a fundamental part in the structuring of the personality, and in the orientation of
human desire.' The 'structuring of the personality,
and the orientation of human desire' means that what
they call 'the different types of relation between the
three points of the triangle' – the child and the two
parents – 'are destined to be internalized and to survive in the structure of the personality'. One's early
Oedipal relations, however changeable and kaleido-
scopic, are a kind of repertoire of possible relations
that are the abiding feature of one's life. So one carries
over into adult life the knowing who or what one
wants with the associated dawdling and evasions and
also a kind of counterlife, or parallel life, in which,
because there are no substitutes for the parents, one
has no idea what or who one wants, radically orientated and radically disorientated at the same time.

In post-Oedipal life one can love and like and

desire all sorts of people and things and ideas, but in parallel-Oedipal life one is extremely picky, or what we call passionate. In post-Oedipal life one notices more; in Oedipal life one is very focused. But, of course, all loving and liking and desiring has an echo of the first Oedipal forms, and so even when we are post-Oedipal we will be inclined to dawdle. But we should not fall into believing that the Oedipal thing is the real thing, because that is the fundamental super-ego command, you must love your parents above all others, thou shall worship no other God. The 'lost' and the 'found' were theological terms before they had psychological currency. So if 'Losing and Being Lost Again' refers to the paper by Anna Freud it is also worth remembering that psychoanalysis is one of the languages that returned to the big themes – what Robert Frost called 'the larger excruciations' – of losing and being lost, with no use for God, or the idea of God. What can losing and being lost mean, what can losing and being lost be redescribed as in a secular context, in the absence of a God? In a human life everything can be lost but everything cannot be found. In other words, once you take one essential figure out of the story of losing and being lost – once you take out the omniscient, the omnipotent figure, the Creator – the story is quite different. There is, for example, the possibility of irredeemable loss, and the question of what it is to be found, or what it would be now not to be found (who is it, one might ask, that hasn't found one?). And there is the question of what it is to lose something, or someone; of what, when one is feeling lost, one is feeling the absence of. What one might depend upon if one didn't depend upon God. What, in the absence of God, played, in the language of Laplanche and Pontalis, the 'fundamental part in the structuring of the personality, and in the orientation of human desire', was inevitably among Freud's questions; and, indeed, among his daughter Anna's questions after he died, Freud having been, as we now know, her analyst. So it is worth looking briefly, by way of introduction, to the prehistory of her remarkable paper 'About Losing and Being Lost', the final version of which was published in 1967.

Anna Freud's biographer Elisabeth Young-Bruehl links the paper to her mourning for her father, who had died in 1939 in London, where they had both taken refuge from the Nazi tyranny. Anna Freud, her biographer tells us, kept records of dreams about her father and about leaving Vienna, along with a set of notes, 'dated December 27, 1942', which she wrote in German but entitled in English 'About Losing and Being Lost'. An essay of this title was drafted in 1948, given as a lecture in 1953 and not published until fourteen years later. It took her, in other words, a long time to finish, and finish with, the paper. And the dreams she had before writing the paper Young-Bruehl sees rightly as being pertinent; as being about the difficulty of losing her father and being lost, in

a certain way, without him. In her dreams, Young-
Bruehl writes,

> Anna Freud again and again found variations on the
> idea that any redirection of her libido would consti-
> tute a betrayal of her father and of her love for him,
> a love that she presents as frankly like a wife's for a
> husband. The betrayal theme and the image of her
> father as a wanderer, 'lost', were ... at the centre of
> her dream-life.

The biography makes it clear just how rejected and
undervalued Anna had felt by her father, how infer-
ior she had felt in his affections compared with her
mother, her aunt and her sister, Sophie. It is intimated
that her dreams after his death reverse this predicament, and Anna has pride of place, the power to betray
her father. The power to make him feel lost, to return
to being the wandering Jew. So the title of the paper
– and, indeed, the difficulty of completion and publication – tells a story: 'About Losing and Being Lost'
spells out in abbreviated form that losing her father
reminded her of how lost he had made her feel, and
how much she had wanted him to recognize this. And
underlying this is the larger, common Oedipal theme,
that feeling lost – as opposed to getting lost – in childhood means not being the chosen one, the special one,
the favourite child; the Oedipal betrayal is the nothing
that comes from not being all.

Freud preferred other women in the family, and Anna, though she did everything for him, could do nothing that would change this. In the family she was inescapably just one among many: nothing special. The only one analysed by her father, the only one who became a psychoanalyst and a pioneer of the so-called 'movement', she was never, in her view, the object of her father's passion. In the secular language of psychoanalysis, 'being lost' means not being specially loved; or, rather, not having one's special love for the parent reciprocated, responded to in kind. It is as if, at least in retrospect, Anna Freud knew what she wanted, her father's special love, and was lost because she didn't get it. In my sense of this, her special love for her father, and her consequent grievance about its being unreciprocated, oriented her desire; it became her map, it took her in certain directions and not others. One way of describing this is that she replaced her love for her father with her grievance against him, and so never renounced her father ('It is typically Jewish,' Freud wrote to his son Ernst on 27 January 1938, 'not to renounce anything and to replace what has been lost'). In these secular terms 'being lost' means losing parental love. So as a child you are not lost until you recognize your dependence on your parents' love, and fear its loss. Being lost and becoming aware of yourself as the object of parental love and desire go together. Lostness turns up in childhood when one becomes, in one's own eyes, the object of someone else's desire. As the subject of her desire the Oedipal child knows where she is; as the object of parental desire she is always potentially lost. As the subject of her own Oedipal desire she will begin to dawdle; as the object of Oedipal desire she will begin to feel herself at worst disappearing, and at best mortally and abjectly wounded. This, at least, is what the biographical material, and its attendant speculations, might lead us to think.

Anna Freud begins her paper, unsurprisingly perhaps, by saying that when it comes to the subject of her essay, 'losing and mislaying objects', her father had got there first. The whole subject, she says, 'came under analytic scrutiny at an early date'; first in 1901 in *The Psychopathology of Everyday Life*, and then more elaborately in Freud's *Introductory Lectures* of 1916, which she quotes. 'Losing and mislaying,' Freud writes:

> are of particular interest to us owing to the many meanings they may have – owing, that is, to the multiplicity of purposes which can be served by these parapraxes. All cases have in common the fact that there was a wish to lose something; they differ on the basis and aim of that wish. We lose a thing when it is worn out, when we intend to replace it with a better one, when we no longer like it, when it originates from someone with whom we are no longer on

good terms or when we acquired it in circumstances
we no longer want to recall.

Implicit in this catalogue of losses is the ruthless, if
unconscious, aggression in such acts; and this is particularly clear if we rephrase Freud's list: we lose interest in people when they are worn out, when we intend
to replace them with a better one, when we no longer
like them, when they come from someone we are not
on good terms with or when we acquired them in circumstances we no longer want to recall. Anna Freud's
interest is in the losses of childhood and the way in
which, as she explains, 'material possessions' represent
either parts of the child's own body or parts of what
she calls 'human love objects'. Because, as she puts it,
'human beings are flexible where their attachments
are concerned', children have 'multiple possibilities for
discharge of their feelings'; when children hate parents or siblings they can attack their toys, when they
separate from parents they cling to loved objects, and
so on. People with 'obsessional characters' are unable
to throw anything away as a reaction formation against
their murderous impulses. 'Losing things is the exception rather than the rule,' she writes, because however
ambivalent we may be, we want to hold on to the
objects we love. From her psychoanalytic point of
view, when we lose something we have unconsciously
got rid of it; consciously we are the victim, unconsciously we are the aggressor.

Losing means hating; feeling lost, for the child, means feeling hated, or unprotected by love. And Anna Freud is able to make psychoanalysis sound like common sense: 'children feel secure, happy and content while they are loved by their parents, and they become insecure, unhappy and hurt in their narcissism if this love is withdrawn, or diminished or changed into aggression'. The difference, as Anna Freud intimates, between adults and children, is that adults are freer to get rid of things and people; the child can't get rid of his body or his parents, or his siblings, even though he may go through periods of wanting to rid himself of them. The child can lose his way, but his way is always back to the parents; growing up means going back to your parents via an increasing number of objects, and in ever longer radii. The child knows where he wants to go even if he doesn't always know the way. Getting lost for the child means, either through aggression or incestuous desire, losing his way, temporarily getting rid of the parents or avoiding the parents; or it means loss of parental love. And for Anna Freud, in this paper, it is the parents' feelings about the child that are the heart of the matter: 'It is only when parental feelings are ineffective or too ambivalent, or when their aggression is more effective than their love, or when the mother's emotions are temporarily engaged elsewhere, that children not only feel lost, but, in fact, get lost.' The child feels lost, or gets lost, when, for whatever reason, the child falls out of the parents' mind. It is common sense that the child would feel lost if the parents are otherwise engaged; but it is psychoanalytic sense that the child might then get lost, and cast himself, as it were, as the lost object; he has become both what the parents seem to want him to be, and a reminder to the parents of what they are making him feel. The child, feeling unloved, identifies with lost objects, and starts losing things, including himself. These children – some of whom Anna Freud observed in her work with separated children during wartime – then play both parts in the forlorn double act of losing and being lost. 'By being chronic losers,' she writes, 'they live out a double identification, passively with the lost objects which symbolize themselves, actively with the parents whom they experience to be as neglectful, indifferent and unconcerned towards them as they themselves are towards their possessions.' When we lose something we are ourselves lost; when we are lost there is something we are at a loss about. But the obverse of this is that being loved means knowing where we are, which is itself an odd idea; or, rather, a theological idea. When we have the experience of knowing where we are, of not feeling lost, we are feeling loved. Parental love, in this quasi-redemptive picture, orientates us; it gives us a map.

And yet implicit in Anna Freud's developmental model is the renouncing of parental love, the so-called resolution of the Oedipus complex in which the child moves on from the parents to more viable objects of desire. Her paper says, explicitly – and of a piece with Young-Bruehl's speculations about her relationship with her father – that without parental love the child is lost, and loses things. But it says nothing about the necessary moving on from the need for parental love; and this may indeed be a need that is never extinguished. A rather literal reading of this paper might lead one to conclude that Anna Freud believed that children need not feel lost if they are sufficiently loved by their parents, and that adults can only feel lost because their parents' love is no longer sufficient. The reassuring version of this story would be that parental love is replaced by the love of someone else. And yet, of course, adults can't and don't love each other in the way parents love children. In Anna Freud's view, as a child one need not feel lost, as an adult one can only feel lost; indeed in her language the capacity to feel lost might be a developmental achievement.

For those, of course, who find ego-psychology and object relations unendearing (those who, for short-hand, we can call Lacanians) the whole notion of knowing where or who one is – or believing that knowing where one is is akin to knowing who one is – is to miss the point of psychoanalysis. It is not Anna Freud's way to idealize unknowing; and in her plain style – she is rather like Kafka in the way she can write so straightforwardly about astoundingly disturbing

and enigmatic matters – the oddest things turn up.
She concludes her paper 'About Losing and Being
Lost' writing about the undead, about the spirits of
dead people that appear in ghost stories, and the lost
and wandering souls who, she says, 'are depicted as
being unable to rest in their burial places and con-
demned instead to wander aimlessly, especially at
night-time, when they moan, sigh and complain, and
beseech the living to help them find release'. Of
course, the voices that can't be buried are the stuff of
psychoanalysis, the hauntings that make us want by
wanting something from us. This gothic horror picture of repression – the unburiable, wandering aimlessly, moaning, sighing, complaining and demanding
– is weirder when it turns up in such sober quasi-
scientific prose. We could think, for example, that
these lost souls might represent a not-so-veiled picture of her and her paper's haunting by her dead
father; but it might also be a picture of what leaving
the parents might feel like, of what it is to feel lost as
an adult, haunted by the memory of parental love and
the knowledge that it is irretrievable. Lost souls,
which we may think of as the dead parents:

> are pitiable rather than threatening and uncanny rather
> than outright frightening. They are 'poor' since they
> symbolize the emotional impoverishment felt by the
> survivor. They are 'lost' as symbols of object loss. That
> they are compelled to 'wander' reflects the wandering

and searching of the survivors' libidinal strivings which have been rendered aimless, i.e., deprived of their former goal. And finally we understand their 'eternal rest' can be achieved only after the survivors have performed the difficult task of dealing with their bereavement and of detaching their hopes, demands and expectations from the image of the dead.

This is what it might feel like when the parents are dead as objects of desire; when, as Anna Freud puts it, 'the wandering and searching of the survivors' libidinal strivings ... have been rendered aimless'. This is a life with no fixed address, with no inevitable, unavoidable destination. The person who leaves his parents needs a map of a place that doesn't exist. Even though he may find and be found he will be to all intents and purposes lost; fundamentally lost, as it were. He may find an object of desire and get lost in its pursuit, dawdle out of anxiety, out of ambivalence, but this will be as close as he can get to recovering from the experience of being ineluctably at a loss. Because the adult, unlike the child, has nowhere to go – nowhere preordained where he goes – he has to go somewhere; because he is now aimless he has to take some kind of aim. This is the goodbye that Anna Freud's paper ends on. Adults are people who keep trying to sustain the illusion that they are not lost, not aimless. Lost to our parents in growing up we are lost souls. People who are lost need a map, virtually any map.

When the critic Frederick Jameson was asked in an interview the mesmerizing question 'Where does "hyperspace" come into the spatial argument?', he said, among other things:

> What is striking about the new urban ensembles around Paris ... is that there is absolutely no perspective at all. Not only has the street disappeared (that was already the task of modernism) but all profiles have disappeared as well. This is bewildering and I use existential bewilderment in this new postmodern space to make a final diagnosis of the loss of our ability to position ourselves within this space and cognitively map it.

I don't know how to understand this kind of grandiose emblem-making, these portentous signs-of-the-times; but for me, in the context of this essay, Jameson is describing something akin to Anna Freud's version of our afterlife as adults, whether or not this is our afterlife as postmodern adults. After childhood, Anna Freud intimates, there is absolutely no perspective at all (in actuality the parents are no basis, no guide for what will follow or replace them). In their existential bewilderment − outside the orbit of the parents' love and its vagaries − adults, post-children, lose their ability to position themselves within this new space and are cognitively unable to map it. The so-called resolution of the Oedipus complex – more ordinarily called leaving home – is finding ways of persuading ourselves that we are not irredeemably lost. The one thing the family can't prepare you for is life outside the family.

On Getting Away with It

When I think of what sort of person I would most like
to have on retainer, I think it would be a boss.

Andy Warhol, *The Philosophy of Andy Warhol*

If guilt is the psychoanalytic word for *not* getting
away with it, what is the psychoanalytic word for
getting away with it? In the psychoanalytic story of
our lives people are always ambivalent and transgressive, whatever else they are; and these predispositions
raise, by implication, the issue of getting away with
something, of avoiding what are deemed to be the
inevitable consequences of certain actions. So if the
human subject, as described by psychoanalysis, is a
split subject, in conflict, by definition, with himself
and others, then getting away with it – harming those
you love, desiring forbidden objects, letting yourself
and others down, sacrificing your desire – is not an
option. There is no truthful, no realistic, description
in the language of psychoanalysis for getting away
with it. And yet, of course, psychoanalysis also urges
us to take our wishes seriously, to read them as dis-

guised formulations of unconscious desire. And there is perhaps no stronger wish – beginning, of course, in childhood – than the wish to get away with things. It is worth wondering therefore what the wish to get away with it is really a wish for; and of course it may be different in each instance.

One of the most interesting things about wishful fantasies and the narratives they provide is where they stop. Of course, they couldn't include all the possible consequences of the gratified wish but they are often surprisingly abbreviated; curtailed all too soon, as if to say: where will it all end? Or, the story of satisfaction is the story we don't know how to tell. In the wishful fantasies of getting away with the prohibited thing we seem to know about the experience we won't have, the experience avoided by the act of getting away with it. If I get away with it, it is as if I know somewhere in myself what it is that I have got away with. I seem to know a great deal about an experience I haven't had. I remember asking a seventy-year-old man who had come to see me whether he had children and he smiled and said, 'No, I managed to get away with it.' When I asked him what he imagined he had got away with he gave me an elaborate and not unfamiliar account of the general inconvenience of having children; he seemed, in a certain sense, immensely authoritative and informed about just how difficult children can be. When I asked him how he knew so much about an experience he hadn't had he said – I thought rather shrewdly – 'Only people who don't have children know what it's really like.' When he said this I was reminded of Winnicott's remark that only a man knows what it's like to be a woman, and only a woman knows what it's like to be a man.

There is, clearly, a kind of knowledge borne of the absence of experience. It often tends towards cliché and omniscience – there is no language more clichéd than the language of the omnipotent – but there is also a freedom to imagine in it. So we might imagine, for example, that a child who gets away with stealing something from a friend – the child, that is to say, who is not caught – knows more about punishment than the one who is found out. And what he knows more about is his super-ego; the language, the severity, the obscenity of the self-punisher he calls up by his act. What he doesn't know about is the experience of being punished and whatever else by the adults, by his peers, by his friend. He might say – I think probably would say – that he knows more about the experience he hasn't had, because he has been able to imagine it. Reality hasn't muscled in and pre-empted the immediacy of his fantasy life. Getting away with it, in other words, gives us the opportunity to consider the senses in which we know more about the experiences we don't have than the experiences we do have.

I know more about being punished by not being punished; I know more about sexuality by never

having sexual experiences with other people. What
is the more that I know? In masturbation, one might
say, it is as if I have got away with having sex without
having to have sex. Perhaps we should take more
seriously than we often do how long we spend in our
lives not having sexual experiences but being, as we
say, full of fantasies; knowing more about what we
might want than about what we can have. An adolescent state of mind is one in which we get away with
being a child and get away with being an adult. Getting away with it – at least in fantasy – may be about
not having to face the consequences; but how can
you face the consequences if you don't and couldn't
know what they are? The phrase 'getting away with
it' makes us face what the phrase 'facing the consequences' might mean. It is realistic to think that if
you have unprotected sex you may conceive a child
or get a sexually transmitted disease; but you can't
know, in the omniscient sense of knowing, what that
would be like for you. The fantasy of getting away
with it, I want to suggest, is not only an excessive
knowingness; it can also be a way of phrasing the possibility that you don't know the consequences of your
actions; a wish not to assume what the gratification
of your wishes might entail. Don't wish too hard or
you'll get what you want means: don't be the false
prophet of your own desire; don't get bamboozled
by your culture – by your upbringing and education
– into being an expert in cause and effect. When I

think, calmly or feverishly, 'I could get away with this,' I am not only giving myself permission, I am also imagining that one thing doesn't always lead to another that I know about. When I imagine getting away with it I am not assuming, consciously, that my act will have no consequences; I am, at best, just assuming it won't have the predictable consequences. It is worth wondering whether some desires are made possible, made riskable, only when sponsored by the fantasy of getting away with it. 'I won't be punished' is both a fear and a wish. Because the other thing getting away with it brings up, or brings on, are the authorities; if you get away with it, does that mean the authorities don't really love you, don't really care about their rules, are in fact quite unable to enforce their rules, are secretly complicit with your breaking them – in short, are not all that they are cracked up to be, cracked up to be by you and yours? If you get away with it is God impotent, absent or negligent? Cynical, or just biding His time, letting you sweat and boast, but leaving you unsure? After all, when do you know, when do you really know, that you have got away with it, that you can finally relax (if getting away with it is just the illusion of getting away with it then you haven't got away with it, you have just protracted the torture, deferred the moment of (punitive) truth)? Or perhaps God is merciful, or sympathetic, or thinks you deserve time out, or time off, or whatever He can do with time to make it kinder. Whichever it is, getting away with it is going to make you think, perhaps like nothing else, about the authorities. They are never more present than when you seem to have slipped their attention. When I am having the all too common fantasy of getting away with it I am thinking about the rules, and how they work and if they work, and what happens to me if they don't.

Sartre tells a story about a young married couple who each morning have breakfast together, then the wife kisses her husband goodbye and sits by the window all day, crying, until he returns; then she perks up. The psychologically minded, Sartre intimates, would say that this young woman is suffering from a separation anxiety; that she is, as some of us might say now, anxiously attached. But in Sartre's view they are wrong because this woman is in fact suffering from a fear of freedom. When her husband goes out she can do, in a sense, whatever she wants – and it is this that terrifies her. The thought of being able to get away with it – the possibility of that – paralyses her. What Sartre doesn't say – probably because it is a mixture of too banal, too bourgeois and too psychoanalytic – is that she may be terrorized by her guilt; her husband's absence leaves her at the mercy, one might say, of her super-ego. From a psychoanalytic point of view – in psychoanalytic language – we have to wonder not whether it would be possible not to feel guilty, but how is it possible, what would it sound like, not to be stifled by guilt? If it didn't sound too pragmatic, too anti-psychoanalytic, the question might be: what, if anything can be done with, or to, guilt? Getting away with it, as a wishful fantasy, is a way of imagining doing something to the super-ego that would make desire seem bearable, that would make pleasure seem pleasurable. Phrases like 'modifying the super-ego' sound plausible only because they sound reasonable. The super-ego as we have construed it may not be the kind of thing, the kind of voice, that can have things like modification done to it. What is to be done that getting away with it might be pointing us in the direction of, consciously and unconsciously?

If the question is: what is it about your life that interests you? – and symptoms, as it were, take the matter out of our hands by forcing our attention (a symptom being whatever it is you can't stop thinking about but would prefer not to) – then the symptom of not having been punished is of particular interest. If you are troubled by not having been punished for something then you might say you are being punished because it preys on your mind as guilt. And yet it is surprisingly common for patients to remember from childhood misdemeanours that went unpunished. These incidents – many of which at face value seem, even to the person confessing, rather minor – seem to have acquired a disproportionate amount of guilt. Of course, a lot of the mischief and delinquency of childhood and adolescence goes unpunished; and yet, for some people, it is the unpunished acts that stay to haunt them. The irony of these predicaments is that punishment, of course, is no longer really available; and yet something is being sought in their being kept as secrets, and their being confessed to in analysis. And often these apparently trivial confessions will be prefaced by the admission that the patient has never told anyone before. It seems to me that often what is being reported on in these moments is an uncompleted action; there was an experience the patient missed having, and it is called punishment. I think we need to bear in mind that 'punishment' is also the word we use, and the thing we do, that brings certain acts to their supposed conclusions; it gives them a sense of an ending. It confirms a cause-and-effect story; it narrows the consequences of actions. If you get away with it, for however long, you are on the open road of unpredictable consequence.

As we know, people, ourselves included, can speak with immense conviction about what is missing in our lives, about the experiences we haven't or aren't having; and about what our lives would be like were we to have them. What is unusual about these not-having-been-punished experiences from childhood – those times when we got away with it, and which stayed with us; these miniature death-of-God experiences when we were abandoned to our transgressions – is that people often have a very limited sense of how their lives would have been better if the requisite, appropriate thing had happened. If I could get the house, the job, the woman or man of my dreams, I can speak at length about how my life would be better. And over time people begin to have a sense, in psychoanalysis, of how their lives might have been different without the deprivations of their childhood. The memories of getting away with it, in childhood and adolescence, are more bluntly enigmatic. If you get away with it, what exactly is the experience you haven't had, given the experience you have had over all these years is a more or less severe private guilt? Indeed, in this scenario guilt might be construed, might be experienced, as a refuge, a retreat, a substitute, a something you had instead of another experience you might have had.

On the straightforward confessional model, or even the less straightforward sadomasochistic model, you could say that external punishment, or at least external acknowledgement – being found out – would have freed you from the burden of guilt and enabled you to void it, to evacuate it by some kind of penitence and reparation. It was a mistake, an error, a falling short of an ideal, and it could have been in some sense recognized as such, and corrected. When someone admits to such things in analysis they want to bring their getting away with it to an end. A patient describes in quite lurid detail how, as a ten-year-old

child, she stole a friend's gloves and buried them
in the back garden; she describes it with such trepidation and terror that you might think – and we,
as analysts, would think – that she had, at least unconsciously, committed a terrible crime. But the terribleness of the crime has been subsumed for her
by the terribleness of having never been caught.
She left a mystery in the world; her friend's gloves
were lost unaccountably and even though the world
may have mostly forgotten them this sixty-three-
year-old woman has not. The world went on making sense for her because she knew how it had
happened; but everyone else involved was left with
what she called 'a hole in the net'. I said to her that
whatever else was going on she had wanted other
people to have the experience that she had had of
things (and people) unaccountably disappearing. She
replied, 'Yes, but I got away with it, because the
gloves hadn't unaccountably disappeared, I had disappeared them!' The experience she couldn't let herself have – the experience we might say that she
couldn't bring within the orbit of her omnipotence
– was of nobody making things happen; of some
things, perhaps the most significant things, happening beyond human agency.

When you get away with it only you know that
the world has changed; you have changed the world
without letting it know. Indeed, if you let it know
it wouldn't have changed. Getting away with it, as a

child and as an adolescent, is a form of radical privacy; and even if you get away with it with accomplices, you are living a version of a private language. You know the crucial thing, the essential fact; you are not the person supposed to know, you are the person who *knows*. Getting away with it, in other words, is an experiment in privacy; it is a conscious solitude with an unconscious backdrop. The person who gets away with it is hyper-conscious of one thing – as in most symptoms – but unconscious of much else.

What I am interested in here is the person's unconscious experience of getting away with it; how, one might say, it makes them live. Because whatever else they are doing, or have been doing, they have been living as if they have got away with something. They are living with an experience – the possibility of an experience – that they have never had. Bringing these things up in analysis is an attempt to find out what the missing experience is assumed to be. The person has a completed narrative – a set of potentially completed narratives – that they are unconscious of. Their imaginations have had to do the work that reality failed to do for them. If reality had intervened, if they had been caught – in itself an interesting phrase – something might have been pre-empted or foreclosed. Or, to change the emphasis slightly, does the young person who gets away with it know more or less about guilt than the person who doesn't? We will, of course, never know, at least in their lifetimes from those who were determined to get away with it, what the guilt experience was like for them: did getting away with it make them bolder or more timid, more ruthless or less; did it make them fans of honesty, or secretly amused by the authorities? We will never know unless they tire of getting away with it; unless, for some reason, as with the patients I mentioned, a time comes when it seems essential to speak about the experience of getting away with it, which, in itself, brings that experience to an end, in its terminal and irrevocable breach of a hard-won and often hard-worn privacy.

What does the adult in analysis, insofar as one can generalize, want from such belated admissions? What is being asked for? That, certainly, is one of the questions being asked in such confessions; and partly because, as the patient usually knows in some part of his mind, the analytic setting is neither a toilet, nor a confessional, but something else altogether.

One of the things that has usefully reconfigured our writing of psychoanalytic theory now is our unavoidable acknowledgement that we can't confidently, any more, make generalizations across cultures, religions, genders, or even perhaps families. All psychoanalytic theorizing has to have now, as a coda, the question: for whom could these sentences be pertinent or useful? Of course, this cuts both ways: because we never know exactly who we are talking about now, we can also be more wildly speculative, and just see who, if anyone, picks it up. I raise this here because getting away with it is so particularly pertinent to immigrant experience, or people trying to live lives they want in oppressive political regimes. The question for these people is: what can I get away with? – a question we are more likely to associate with adolescents or criminals. How can I get away with living according to the things I believe in a society which either outrightly outlaws these practices – Muslim children in France, for example, have by law to obey secular dress codes – or is prejudiced against them? In these contexts what we might call getting away with it can be a matter of life or death; or a matter of ethical life or death. As honourable psychoanalysts in Germany in the 1930s we would not presumably be turning in our Jewish patients and colleagues to the Nazis. In other words, what we, in a psychoanalytic way, would think of as the childhood wish – or the wish beginning in childhood – to get away with it turns out, obviously, to have complicated and sometimes untrackable repercussions. What is going to be the fate of someone who, broadly speaking, feels unable, or unwilling, to get away with things? For whom the whole notion of getting away with things – which might, by displacement, seem to be rather trivial things – is unbearable, something they would prefer not to have in their personal repertoire?

By way of an answer to my question – what are people asking for in analysis by making their belated admissions of often minor misdemeanours? – there is one obvious consideration, though it is not often obvious to the person making the admission, and that is: what has made guilt so unbearable to them, what is their personal history of this essential feeling such that they need to invite in another person to their predicament? And then there is the question – the answers to which are partly unconscious, and will differ in each case, and at each time – of what exactly is wanted from the analyst. What is the experience they haven't had – the missing experience, as it were – that, it is imagined, will complete or at least continue the story of the crime? What is being asked for is the provision not of the missing experience necessarily, but of an account of what the missing experience might have been felt to be. There was something they got away with, and something they got away without. What can be done in analysis – and it will of course be partly guess-work, the best kind of work psychoanalysts do – is to consider the possibilities and what they might have led to. You cannot of course supply missing experiences, but you can describe what they might have been – what might have been wanted, or feared, or both – and how that might have made the person's life different. And something in all this describing may be useful material for a possible future. We can never be quite sure when the possibility for an experience is over; wanting to mourn missed opportunities is sometimes an attempt to foreclose this unknowable future. Getting away with it, whatever else the phrase portends, is a way of talking about unexpectable experience.

Forms of Inattention

You know how you know when someone's
telling lies? you said. They
get their story right every time, down to the
last word.

Whereas when they tell the truth it's never the
same twice. They
reformulate.

Ciaran Carson, 'The Shadow'

I Arbus's Freaks

… but we have the right to be seduced.

Dave Hickey, *The Invisible Dragon*

If it is too often said about Diane Arbus that she
photographs freaks it does at least suggest, at its most
minimal, that we know what normal people are like,
what people look like when they are not odd. It is

reassuring to be reminded not only that we are not all freaks, but also that we know a freak when we see one. There are, of course, points of view, angles from which we can all look like freaks to ourselves; and Arbus, as we shall see, is unusually eloquent about this and about how the camera is, as it were, good at picking up the unwanted perspective. But the enthusiastic unease that Arbus's work generates, and the pleasure we take from her work, must have something to do with our wondering what it must be to be people like that; and, by the same token, what it must be to be people like us, who are not freaks like that but for some reason – and Arbus was herself exercised by this – are fascinated by freaks like that. Indeed, we want pictures and exhibitions of them; and we want something from representations of them that we mostly don't want from them in person. Pictures of these people – or, rather, Arbus's unique way of not turning a blind eye – satisfy something in us. She has not, it should be noted, created a fashion for her subject matter, but for her photographs. Arbus's photographs, whatever else they do, create a kind of vicarious sociability with people we suspect we mostly wouldn't be able to get on with.

One of the many interesting things about photography as a relatively new art form is that photographers talking and writing about their work is also a relatively new genre. And Arbus, it seems to me, was unusually eloquent as well as unusually keen and willing to articulate something about what she thought she was doing, mindful as people usually are that words for pictures is a peculiar form of exchange. When Arbus speaks of her work she often enough talks of photography as a form of sociability: 'some pictures are tentative forays without your even knowing it'. The camera, of course, gives the photographer something to do with other people, and the camera is like a safe lead, a 'licence', as she calls it, into the unpredictable. Who you can and can't be with, for Arbus, is bound up with what you can and can't know about people. As a certain kind of modern artist she thinks of intentions as passwords that get you what you never expected; and she locates the mystery that matters most to her, her preferred mystery, in the unfamiliar (the family being the place where unfamiliarity begins). 'I remember one summer,' she writes:

> I worked a lot in Washington Square Park. It must have been about 1966. The park was divided. It has these walks, sort of like a sunburst, and there were these territories staked out. There were young hippie-junkies down one row. There were lesbians down another, really tough, amazingly hard-core lesbians. And in the middle were winos ... They were like the first echelon, and the girls who came from the Bronx to become hippies would have to sleep with the winos to get to sit on the other part with the junkie-hippies. It was really remarkable.

And I found it very scary. I mean, I could become a
nudist, I could become a million things. But I could
never become that, whatever all those people were.
There were days I just couldn't work there, and then
there were days I could. And then, having done it
a little, I could do it more. I got to know a few of
them. I hung around a lot. They were a lot like
sculptures in a funny way. I was very keen to get
close to them, so I had to ask to photograph them.
You can't get that close to somebody and not say a
word, although I have done that.

I take this to be a kind of parable of Arbus as a
photographer. There is well-known biographical
material that would seem to make a certain sense of
this, to do with Arbus's recollected sense of being
secluded, segregated in the affluent Jewish family she
grew up in. 'One of the things I suffered from as
a kid,' she said, 'was I never felt adversity. I felt con-
firmed in a sense of unreality which I could feel as
unreality, and the sense of being immune was, ludi-
crous as it seems, a painful one . . . the world seemed
to belong to the world. I could learn things but they
never seemed to be my own experience.' The gist
of the recollection is her strong sense that there
was somewhere else she needed to get to, some other
kind of experience, some necessary illness that she
was immune to. It is unlikely that she never felt
adversity as a child, but likely that she might have felt

in retrospect that she didn't get the adversity she
wanted. In Washington Square Park in 1966 the world
seems to belong to the world again, she doesn't belong
to it. And what she's interested in in the groups she
observes is how people who are so separated can
get together: 'the girls who came from the Bronx to
become hippies would have to sleep with the winos
to get to sit on the other part with the junkie-hippies'.
And Arbus is quite clear that here she has reached her
limit, the horizon of her ambition: 'I could become a
million things. But I could never become that, whatever all those people were.' But what you can't become
you can photograph; you can get close to. And the
way to get close to them is to ask them for something: 'I was very keen to get close to them, so I had
to ask to photograph them. You can't get that close
to somebody and not say a word, although I have
done that.' If you ask someone for a photograph of
themselves you are asking them to give you one, not
to let you take one. Arbus – for some reason she
doesn't need to articulate – wants to get close to these
people 'whatever all those people were', and the way
is to ask to photograph them: words for pictures. But
in this process – and I think the parable is calculated,
wittingly or unwittingly, to make us wonder about
this – what does that make the photograph? If her
work, if the camera, is an ice-breaker – a way of having something to do with these people who she could
never become – what is the picture a picture of? If we

take Arbus at her word, the pictures are of an impossible aspiration: 'I could never become that, whatever all those people were.' They are records, or reminders, so to speak, of a thwarted closeness; of where sociability stops. You can't be with these people; and this is where the photography, the work, comes in.

Sometimes Arbus starts from the diametrically opposed position, with no affinity, no longing, as though alienation from, or the irrelevance of, the subject matter was the precondition of the work. 'The Chinese have a theory,' she writes, 'that you pass through boredom into fascination, and I think it's true. I would never choose a subject for what it means to me or what I think about it. You've just got to choose a subject, and what you feel about it, what it means, begins to unfold if you just plain choose a subject and do it enough.' In Washington Square Park she starts with the fascination; here she ends up with the fascination through apparently arbitrary choice and dogged persistence. But in this latter formulation the photograph is far more, and far more obviously, significant; it is the revelation of feeling and meaning. The photograph gets you closer not to the object, but to the photographer's unfolding apprehension of the object. As ever with Arbus, closeness is the issue; and it is presumably not insignificant that so many of her photographs are so close up, and quite often of people one mostly wouldn't want to be that close to; at least in so-called real life.

'Nothing is ever the same as they said it was,' Arbus says. 'It's what I've never seen before that I recognize.' What other people say distances you; if it's 'what I've never seen before that I recognize' we have to assume that this is because 'they' prevented her with their words from seeing the thing that mattered to her. '[T]hey' have kept her away, immune, unreal, and her project, the New — 'what I've never seen before' — becomes the desired; it represents, it becomes symbolically equated with, the necessary thing from which she has been somehow excluded. Her question, I think, or rather her dilemma, is, how much does she want to know, how close does she want to get to whatever it is she believes she has been excluded from? Arbus starts from a position of exclusion; the people in Washington Square Park, like the arbitrarily chosen subject, are nothing to do with her. Arbus is never sure whether she is interested in the experience of exclusion — and her so-called freaks are, by definition, the excluded that she is including — or whether she is interested in finding out exactly what it might be that she is excluded from, which is what her so-called freaks make us think about. Becoming obsessed with exclusion can become a way, perhaps *the* way, of not thinking about what it might be that one is excluded from. So when Arbus (a bit too famously) says, 'A photograph is a secret about a secret. The more it tells you the less you know,' she is both making a distinction between showing and telling which photographs draw to our attention, and also giving us her potted theory of secrecy. What a photograph apparently tells you is what you don't need to know; that in photography the explicit is always misleading; and that photography, at least in Arbus's version, is a peculiarly intent form of secrecy. A 'secret about a secret' means that what is being kept a secret is that there is a secret. Photographs, unlike photographers, can't actually speak; and a 'secret about a secret' is as good a definition of the unconscious as one is likely to get. But a 'secret about a secret' is two degrees of separation. Arbus is not saying that she knows what the secret is; she is just saying she knows that what is being kept secret in the photograph is that there is a secret.

The photograph, or, rather, in Arbus's words about the photograph, has something to show us, if not tell us, not about odd people, but about how odd we are about closeness and exclusion. Many of her photographs have a baroque longing in them. And many of her remarkable statements about her work have something to say about the dread and the draw of being left out. 'Lately I've been struck,' she says, 'with how I really love what you can't see in a photograph. An actual physical darkness. And it's very thrilling for me to see darkness again.' To see darkness is to see what you can't see, and what you can't see through. In Arbus's photographs the thrill of being left out contends with the dread. It would be terrible to believe that there is nothing to be left out

of. What, we are invited to think about Arbus's photographs, are the so-called freaks in her pictures left
out of, and what is it about this that is at once so
poignant and so horrifying for us? Or, to put it a little more glibly, who is left out of what? If we so
much want to look at Arbus's pictures of freaks, what
are we feeling excluded from?

The story Arbus wants to tell us explicitly about
freaks – that is to say, in words rather than in photographs – is that she is envious of them. 'Freaks was a
thing I photographed a lot,' she says, not wary of using
either word:

> It was one of the first things I photographed and it
> had a terrific kind of excitement for me. I just used
> to adore them. I still do adore some of them. I don't
> quite mean they're my best friends but they made
> me feel a mixture of shame and awe. There's a qual-
> ity of legend about freaks. Like a person in a fairy
> tale who stops you and demands that you answer a
> riddle. Most people go through life dreading they'll
> have a traumatic experience. Freaks were born with
> their trauma. They've already passed their test in life.
> They're aristocrats.

This is characteristically shrewd and unsettling,
both in its blitheness and in its gravity. Like some of
her best photographs it's somewhere between a comedy routine – 'I just used to adore them. I still do

adore some of them. I don't quite mean they're my best friends' – and an existential fable. They are at once both unreal – things, legends, people in fairy tales, aristocrats – and very intensely real: they've got their trauma in first, they've 'passed their test in life', they are aristocrats. They are, one could say, from a slightly different angle, or 'corner', to use Arbus's word; a bit like Jews, born members of the aristocracy of trauma. And what is striking about Arbus's account is just how explicit she is about the erotics, the fantasies, in being a fan. There is a terrific kind of excitement, adoration, shame, awe. And the lives of her freaks, in her version, are constituted by what they are excluded from. Because they are born with their trauma they are born with the very thing that will separate them out from others. That's where they start from, not what they have to go in search of, as Arbus did in Washington Square Park. It is as though their test in life, *the* test in life, for Arbus, is what you make of your exclusion, or of the thing that excludes you. The camera, one can see in Arbus's Washington Square Park parable, is the object that at once includes you and excludes you. But Arbus, quite rightly, is keen to remind us always that the photograph is not in any simple sense its subject; it is its so-called subject represented, recognized in a quite different medium. And clearly to talk about photography is to talk about this difference in new ways because photography appears to be so effortlessly mimetic. 'What I'm trying to describe,' she says, 'is that it's impossible to get out of your skin into some-body else's. And that's what all this is a little bit about. That somebody else's tragedy is not the same as your own.' Perhaps the thing one is most left out of is other people's traumas, other people's tragedies. You don't need a photograph of a freak, or indeed to pho-tograph a freak, to tell you that you are not a freak yourself. So what, to ask the pragmatic question, are Arbus's photographs of freaks for? Why photograph them, and why photograph them like that? 'Freaks was a thing I photographed a lot. It was one of the first things I photographed and it had a terrific kind of excitement for me.' One of the first things, that is, after the fashion models she and her husband photo-graphed in the 1940s. There is possibly a suggestion here that freaks were Arbus's way into her own kind of photography. So it is worth wondering, by way of conclusion, what that was a way into.

Arbus describes becoming fascinated in the 1960s by a blind street performer who, she says, 'lives in an atmosphere as dense and separate as an island with its own sea'. An 'island with its own sea' is indeed a very separate island. If Arbus was drawn to the impossi-bilities of closeness then it is tempting to suggest that her photographs at once both record this impossibil-ity and try to break it down. Eudora Welty remarked that Arbus's work 'totally violates human privacy, and by intention', as though Arbus couldn't bear or, more interestingly, didn't trust the privacy of others. As though privacy was some kind of mystification; as though the opaqueness of ourselves and others was becoming sacralized. Welty was overstressing something – violation tends to be total, no one talks of feeling 'a bit violated' – that is important about Arbus's work. If anything, though, I think it may be truer to say that Arbus's work is more often showing us just how inviolable modern human privacy actually is; however close or close up you get, you never get that close. And that there is something about modern life that generates fantasies of closeness, of intimacy, that are way in excess of human possibility. Secrets can be found out, but privacy cannot be violated because once it is violated it is no longer privacy. The idea of secrecy is the last refuge of romance. It may not be that we have secrets, but that each person sees us differently. It may not be that we are at our most revelatory in our intimacies, but at our most anonymous. These, at least, are the areas that Arbus leads us into when she talks and writes about photography. 'Our whole guise,' she writes, 'is like giving a sign to the world to think of us in a certain way but there's a point between what you want people to know about you and what you can't help people knowing about you.' Other people see us in ways that we cannot anticipate; we cannot know ourselves because we cannot be everyone else in relation to ourselves; and so on.

It is clear from all this just how psychologically minded Arbus is when she talks and writes about photography. And like all good psychological writing it sounds compelling and pertinent; and it is not surprising that Arbus, growing up and working when and where she did, found this kind of language to hand. But this way of talking can take us a long way from the photographs as photographs, especially when someone is as eloquent and canny as Arbus obviously was. The worse your art is, the American poet John Ashbery once remarked, the easier it is to talk about. What I think is truly odd about Arbus's work is not her subject matter, but how difficult it is to resist speaking psychologically about it; or, to put it another way, how difficult it is to conceive of not talking about it in psychological terms. And I don't mean as an alternative to this talking technically. To look at Arbus's photographs without trying to imagine what might be going on inside her subjects; as if, in fact, you couldn't. A person who is as dense and separate as an island with its own sea may not be available for that, and so may be available for something else. For being photographed.

II Celebrating Sebald

There is always hope except when there isn't –
it is everywhere.

Frederick Seidel, 'Sunlight'

'Is literary greatness still possible?' Susan Sontag
asked in 2000: 'Given the implacable devolution of
literary ambition, and the concurrent ascendancy of
the tepid, the glib, and the senselessly cruel as nor-
mative fictional subjects, what would a noble literary enterprise look like now? One of the few answers
available to English-language readers is the work
of W. G. Sebald.' 'When *The Emigrants* appeared
in English in 1996,' her encomium continued, 'the
acclaim bordered on awe ... what seemed foreign
and most persuasive was the preternatural authority
of Sebald's voice; its gravity, its sinuosity, its preci-
sion, its freedom from all undermining or undigni-
fied self-consciousness or irony.' There was palpable
relief – among many people of similar educations –
that great literature could still be written. A voice of
'preternatural authority' seems a little scary, and possibly a little ill-judged given the period of European
history that preoccupied Sebald. But Sontag was
clearly voicing something that was widely felt; the

reviews of Sebald's books as they came out in the 1990s were, even by contemporary standards, unusually enthusiastic.

Indeed, it is difficult to remember a contemporary writer celebrated on quite this scale. There was a virtual consensus: *The Emigrants*, Cynthia Ozick wrote in the *New Republic*, was 'sublime'; for the reviewer in the *Chicago Tribune* it was 'a unique masterpiece'; for the *Spectator* 'an unconsoling masterpiece'; and for Sontag 'an astonishing masterpiece'. It was clearly not enough for the book to be just a masterpiece. *The Rings of Saturn*, to give one more example, was greeted by James Wood in the *Guardian* as 'a great, strange and moving work'. 'Sebald is surely a major European author,' John Murray wrote in the *Independent on Sunday*, who 'reaches the heights of epiphanic beauty only encountered normally in the likes of Proust'. It is perhaps more difficult to be eloquently celebratory than eloquently critical, which is itself interesting, and Sebald's books, as we shall see, have something to say about this. But these blurbs suggest also that Sebald's remarkable books made people want to celebrate his writing in quite extraordinary ways.

There were, of course, dissenting voices: 'One of the most striking developments in English-language publishing in the last five years,' the poet and translator Michael Hoffman wrote in a piece in *Prospect* magazine entitled 'A Chilly Extravagance', 'has been

the extraordinary success of the books of W. G. Sebald.'
'The complete absence of humour, charm, grace,
touch is startling,' he wrote, 'as startling as the fact
that books written without them could enjoy any
sort of success in England.' Sebald's writing, Hoffman claimed, had been 'more often praised than
accurately described', and he attempted to remedy
the situation by going on about Sebald's 'chilly extravagance ... numbed obsessiveness ... the complacency
and lack of urgency in Sebald's academic sleuthing
and the pedantic rosters of his prose catalogues'.
Clearly what disturbs Hoffman is the blizzard of
praise that met Sebald's work. And even if one dis-
agrees with the content of Hoffman's criticism – and
it is surely startlingly wrong to find Sebald's writing
humourless or charmless – he does pick up on an
interesting question: why exactly is Sebald's writing
praised in such effusive ways, and what exactly is
being celebrated? What kind of pleasure do we get
from Sebald's often grim, always melancholic books?
When Bob Dylan was asked on American radio if
he had been surprised by the success of *Blood on the
Tracks*, he said, after a pause, that he didn't know
how people got so much pleasure from so much pain.
It is not news that people get pleasure from pain, but
how they do it is worth considering. And one of the
tasks that such consideration might involve is finding
better descriptions of what it is to celebrate or to
praise.

At the heart of this essay is a simple observation: Sebald's much-celebrated writing has itself very interesting things to say about celebration. Sebald's writing is indeed obsessed with greetings and welcomes, with festivities and the difficulties that attend them, and with celebration as a kind of remembering. In this regard, the responses, our responses, to Sebald's writing appear as puzzling, in their way, as the books themselves. And the puzzle, I think, has partly to do with celebration. 'Surely one of the things that makes it so difficult to write about Sebald,' the critic Eric Santner writes,

> to say anything new or genuinely revelatory about his work, is that he has done so much himself to frame the discourse of his own reception, to provide in advance the terms for critical engagement with the work; his fiction already practises a rather efficient sort of autoexegesis that leaves the critic feeling a certain irrelevance (the posture of awestruck adoration that one finds in so much of the critical literature is, I think, one of the guises such irrelevance assumes).

In Santner's view, Sebald hasn't so much created the taste by which he wants to be judged as already established it – as though all we can really do when we write about Sebald is go on quoting him. But what bothers Santner, as it did Michael Hoffman, is the 'awestruck adoration' of Sebald, as though this in itself tells us something crucial about the writing, about how it works on us. Hoffman intimated that the extravagant celebration of Sebald was a way of overlooking the flaws in the work: 'Sebald's writing has been more often praised than accurately described,' he wrote, as though praise protects us from what might be revealed by further description. Or, to put it slightly differently, and rather more meanly, we might sometimes celebrate when we fear a fault-finding mission coming on. For Santner, the critic's 'awestruck adoration' of Sebald's writing is a kind of solution to 'the critic feeling a certain irrelevance', perhaps feeling he has nothing to add, can't really contribute, doesn't quite know what to say. By implication, then, 'awestruck adoration' gives the critic something to do, keeps a feeling of irrelevance at bay, cures redundancy. For both Hoffman and Santner the adoring praise of Sebald's writing is a solution to something, perhaps a problem posed by (or perceived in) the work. What Sebald is often telling us in his writing is that our solutions reveal the full extent of our problems; that our cures – or our imagined cures – expose the full nature of our suffering rather than making it disappear.

There is a small example at the beginning of *Vertigo* when the narrator, in talking about Stendhal's Italian adventures, enters into the very big subject of what he calls 'the various difficulties entailed in the act of recollection'. 'It was a severe disappointment for Stendhal,' the narrator learns from his notes, when some years ago, looking through old papers, he came across an engraving entitled *Prospetto D'Ivrea* and was obliged to concede that his recollected picture of the town in the evening sun was nothing but a copy of that very engraving. This being so, [Stendhal's] advice is not to purchase engravings of fine views and prospects seen on one's travels since before very long they will displace our memories completely, indeed one might say they destroy them.

This passage may allude to (or simply echo) Walter Benjamin's remark in 'Central Park' that 'the souvenir is the complement to isolated experience. In it is precipitated the increasing self-estrangement of human beings, whose past is inventoried as dead effects.' Sebald, through Stendhal, makes the dilemma more vividly immediate by making it simpler; we buy souvenirs to help us remember, and then what we remember are the souvenirs. Indeed, collecting souvenirs is an attack on memory, as though, unwittingly, we buy souvenirs in order to forget where we have been, to displace our memories; or perhaps we interfere with the workings of memory by trying to fix our memories in souvenirs. If the problem is, how can I remember where I have been? or, more interestingly, how can I remember what I want to remember? then the proposed solution is, buy a souvenir. But what the solution, the souvenir, reveals is the problem of remembering: we can't always remember what we want to remember, and in the ways we want to remember. Indeed, souvenirs reveal just how precarious memory is, how we want to pre-empt its workings, how distrustful we are of it, how we want to destroy it. Souvenirs disclose just how keen we are to forget things, how we can hate memory and want to ruin its works. What do you do with an object of desire? You try to remember it in its absence. But your very ways of remembering it reveal your wish to ablate it, reveal just how elusive, how unpredictable, it is in the way it works on you. The souvenir is not an aide-mémoire; rather, it reminds you how memory itself works, how it can work against you, and how it works beyond your calculation. Our solutions are redescriptions of our problems.

Again, Sebald is exercised by the paradox that only our solutions reveal our problems to us, or the full horror of our problems, Sebald's narrator might say. If a souvenir in some way celebrates an experience – 'extols' it, makes it 'publicly known', 'solemnizes' it, to use *The Oxford English Dictionary* definitions of celebration – what it is celebrating is that one doesn't know what the experience was or even whether one has digested it; in a sense, a souvenir is celebrating the destruction of the memory, but in the guise of its preservation. Celebrations, as anybody who has had a birthday party they didn't want knows (birthdays

being of some significance in Sebald's work), can feel
like rather mixed experiences. Celebration, we can
say – at least from a psychoanalytical point of view
– is an ambivalent act pretending not to be one.

Our solutions show us our problems; our self-
cures – as Sebald often makes patently clear in his
mordantly witty way – bring on and bring out the
real depth of our suffering. *The Rings of Saturn* begins
with, and is born out of, this experience. It is, as often
in Sebald's books, that the narrator is trying to help
himself, walk himself out of what he is suffering
from, and by doing so walks himself straight into it.
The book begins,

In August 1992, when the dog days were drawing to
an end, I set off to walk the country of Suffolk, in
the hope of dispelling the emptiness that takes hold
of me whenever I have completed a long stint of
work. And in fact my hope was realized, up to a
point; for I have seldom felt so carefree as I did then,
walking for hours in the day through the thinly
populated countryside, which stretches inland from
the coast. I wonder now, however, whether there
might be something in the old superstition that certain ailments of the spirit and of the body are particularly likely to beset us under the sign of the Dog
Star. At all events, in retrospect, I became preoccupied not only with the unaccustomed sense of freedom but also with the paralysing horror that had

come over me at various times when confronted
with the traces of destruction, reaching far back into
the past, that were evident even in that remote place.
Perhaps it was because of this that, a year to the day
after I began my tour, I was taken into a hospital in
Norwich in a state of almost total immobility. It
was then that I began in my thoughts to write these
pages.

His mobility ends up immobilizing him. His attempted
cure for the emptiness of finishing a piece of writing
works initially. He is carefree, at least at first, but there
is some implied connection between his 'unaccustomed sense of freedom' and the 'paralysing horror'
that comes over him 'when confronted with the traces
of destruction, reaching far back into the past, that
were evident even in that remote place'. On the one
hand, he simply can't get away from the traces of
destruction, even when he gets away from people;
and on the other hand, it is almost as if his unusual
sense of freedom can't protect him from these traces,
or as if he is even freer to see them. It is not insignificant, though it is done as always in Sebald without
portentousness, that freedom, perhaps our most
highly valued political and personal ideal and aspiration – even when briefly achieved by the solitary
walker – is impotent against the traces of destruction;
it is not that his freedom can't hold at bay just how
destructive even the traces of human destructiveness

are, it is that his freedom is a freedom to see them as
they are. He is in 'a state of almost total immobility'.
Freedom is neither the cure nor a solution to his condition. And just as Sebald's books work like echo
chambers – things are always resonating and return-
ing and coinciding – so towards the end of the book,
when the solitary walker goes to the strange and
rather sinister island of Orfordness, he feels 'at the
same time both utterly liberated and deeply despond-
ent. I had not a single thought in my head.' Being
free is not equated with feeling better – there are
many traces of destructiveness on the island, which
was full of 'military installations'.

Feeling utterly liberated, which is presumably
cause for celebration, turns out to be radically deplet-
ing. Given the references to the war, there may be
echoes in this passage of the liberation of concentration camps in which, once again, celebration becomes
a peculiarly mixed thing. How can we celebrate, or
what are we doing when we celebrate, in a world
that is packed out with traces of destruction that are
only reminders of the ongoing destruction that
Sebald's narrators so relentlessly document? 'To what
it was that I owed thanks for my utterly unexpected
recovery late that winter, or whether thanks is the
right word, I know as little as I know how one gets
through this life,' the character Luisa writes in a
memoir given to the narrator by Max Ferber in *The
Emigrants*. Recovery (at least in English, and, of course,

Sebald is a writer read in English translation) combines remembering and getting better. Sebald's narrators are sceptical about this connection, and indeed about whether 'thanks' is the right word. What is there to celebrate, and what is it to celebrate, when 'confronted with the traces of destruction, reaching far back into the past'? What is celebration a solution to, a self-cure for? These are the much-celebrated Sebald's abiding questions.

Birthdays are important in Sebald's writing for their astrological significance, for the coincidences they provide, and for the celebrations that do and don't occur around them. So his own birthday, celebrated or at least recounted in *After Nature*, is of some interest. One's birthday is the most significant event in one's life in the sense that without it there aren't any other events; and yet the only memory of this significant event exists in the form of other people's accounts. A birthday is thus the celebration of an event that one cannot remember, an event in which one was the only person there who wasn't present. Birthdays, to begin with, are the history one depends upon other people for. As described in *After Nature*, on Sebald's birthday, unsurprisingly perhaps, celebration was tempered by catastrophe, presenting just the kind of absurdist coincidence that Sebald relishes:

At the moment on Ascension Day
of the year forty-four when I was born

the procession for the blessing of the fields
was just passing our house to the sounds
of the fire-brigade band, on its way out
to the flowering May meadows. Mother
at first took this as a happy sign, unaware
that the cold planet Saturn ruled this hour's
constellation and that above the mountains
already the storm was hanging, which soon thereafter
dispersed the supplicants and killed
one of the four canopy bearers.

Two celebrations, Christ's Ascension and Sebald's
birth, were ironically juxtaposed and his mother
naively took that as a happy sign; both were spoiled
by unexpected disaster; to celebrate his birthday is
also to remember the death of one of the canopy bearers. What happened, in this case through no one's
agency, meant that there would always be more to
Sebald's birthday celebrations than the celebration of
his birth. There is, Sebald will often intimate, an ominous excess in celebration, a storm in the offing. 'Benjamin at one point says,' Sebald says in an interview
with Michael Silverblatt, 'that there is no point in
exaggerating that which is already horrific. And from
that, by extrapolation one can conclude that perhaps
in order to get the full measure of the horrific, one
needs to remind the reader of the beatific moments of
life.' The beatific moments in life – and it is a not
insignificant choice of words – remind one what one

has lost or destroyed, or what has been destroyed. The beatific, the making blessed, may be the best way we have to get the full measure of the horrific.

In the account of his birth in *After Nature*, the blessing of the fields leads to the death of one of the canopy bearers. In *The Rings of Saturn*, the 'unaccustomed sense of freedom' brings with it the 'paralysing horror'. Both moments suggest that our celebrations are dark reminders. In Sebald's writing celebration can quite literally portend disaster, as though the celebration itself is the registration of the forthcoming catastrophe. 'Whenever one is imagining a bright future,' he writes in *The Rings of Saturn*, 'the next disaster is just around the corner.' Alternatively, signs of celebration are signs of loss, like the bridal gown made by the bizarre Irish spinster sisters in the same novel, a gown 'made of hundreds of scraps of silk embroidered with silken thread, or rather woven over cobweb-fashion, which hung on a headless tailor's dummy' and which, like all the things the sisters endlessly make and unmake, will never be used. As Penelopes without husbands, or betrayed Miss Havishams, the three sisters in all their literary and mythical allusiveness are reminders of horrific losses and destructions. It is indeed what the objects of celebration (like the wedding gown) allude to, what celebration refers us to, that preoccupies Sebald. Celebrations can help us forget what will happen after the celebrations are over.

Celebration is what we do with the things and

people we value; and the loss and traces of destruction that obsess Sebald in his writing matter only because there are objects of desire, people and things, we do love and value. So to cast suspicion on celebration, to wonder what we may be up to when we are celebrating, might seem like an unusually joyless task; not to celebrate celebration, not to 'praise whatever you can' (in the poet Stephen Dunn's words), is at best against the spirit of the age, and at worst the death of the spirit. And yet Sebald, I think, feels about celebration what he tells Arthur Lubow he feels about metaphysics: 'if one thing interests me it is metaphysics. I am not seeking an answer, I just want to say "this is very odd indeed."' This sounds like the kind of ingenuous exclamation that Wittgenstein – another writer important to Sebald – tends to make in his philosophical inquiries. And as with Wittgenstein, it is not that Sebald has a theory about celebration (or metaphysics) in any sense, but that throughout his writing instances of it keep turning up: situations – like his many arrivals in empty hotels or meetings with people – in which celebration may or may not be the issue; or simply reminders that celebration is one of the things that we do in what he calls, in his lugubrious way, 'our history which is but a long account of calamities'. It is as if he wants to say about celebration, 'this is very odd indeed'.

So if it sometimes seems that a kind of plangent desolation is Sebald's expectable environment, that traces of destruction are everywhere in his landscape, there is also a great deal of avid energy and curiosity in his narrators. Indeed, one thing that confounds them is their undefeatedness. The relentless research and erudition of his narrators – at once a parody of the academic life, and a life-and-death struggle to keep going – is tempered by a reiterated gloom. On his way to Colmar in *The Emigrants* the narrator feels 'a kind of festive good spirits rising with me'; but by the end of the page, seventeen lines later, he is telling us, 'what is certain though is that mental suffering is effectively without end. One may think one has reached the very limit, but there are always more torments to come.' These, one might say, are the kinds of conclusions that Sebald's narrators tend to put their trust in, even if sometimes we can feel that they protest too much. But because the terror and the desolation and the general dismay are taken for granted – and this assumption has an obvious religious and historical provenance – the moments of relief and release can seem like moments of grace or revelation. In the fourth section of *Vertigo* the narrator is on a bus full of local women in the Tyrolean mountains. 'They talked mainly or indeed exclusively,' the narrator writes,

about the never-ending rain, which in many places had already caused whole mountainsides to slide into the valleys. They spoke of the hay rotting in the fields and the potatoes rotting in the ground; of the red-

currants that had come to nothing for the third year
in a row ... As they went on discussing the effects of
the ever-worsening weather, complaining that there
was neither sunlight nor warmth, the scene outside
brightened up, a little at first then more and more.
One could now see the river Inn, its waters meander-
ing through broad stony reaches, and soon beautiful
meadows came into view. The sun came out, the
entire landscape was radiant, and the Tyrolean women
fell silent one after the other and simply looked out at
the miracle passing by. I felt much the same myself ...
the steaming forests and the blue skies above, though
I had come up from the south and had had to endure
the Tyrolean darkness for only a couple of hours,
were like a revelation even to me.

This sudden transfiguration of the landscape was a
revelation even to him, and yet it is evident to the
reader that the narrator of *Vertigo* – like the narrators
of Sebald's other documentary fictions – has himself
been talking 'mainly or indeed exclusively' about the
never-ending rain and destruction of natural life; he
is always haunted by the approaching state of 'after
nature'. But perhaps it is more difficult – or difficult
in a quite different way, as the parable says – to
articulate one's thoughts about the desired object,
the longed-for state, the time, when it comes, that
you have been looking forward to. Like the women
on the bus, the narrator can go on and on talking

about 'the ever-worsening weather', but when the
sun comes out they are struck dumb. It isn't necessarily that words fail them, but that they find themselves
not speaking; it is, as it were, a silent celebration: 'the
Tyrolean women fell silent one after the other and
simply looked out at the miracle passing by'. At least
in the translation this is a different kind of fall; the
commentary stops, the storytelling fades out, and
they start simply to look. And this too, it is intimated,
is a kind of miracle. (The scene from Sebald parallels
a striking pattern in psychoanalytic practice with older
children. They tend to take good experiences with
their parents for granted and talk about grievances.
The frustrations return as articulated unhappiness; the
good things, paradoxically, are not worth talking
about, or there is just nothing to say about them.)

The Tyrolean women, like the narrator, celebrate
the breaking through of the sun in silence; they just
take it in. And that – even though, as always in Sebald,
the scene is entirely convincing – is odd. In this
instance, celebration is silent, grievance and fear are
not. Here the beatific moment is not there 'in order
to get the full measure of the horrific'; indeed, what
is gained from that moment is not articulated. The
solution, the sun, that calls up this silence in the
women renders their suffering unfathomable; in this
instance all we can know is that just looking is the
form the celebration takes. One thing we might infer
from this – though, rightly, no one in the book draws

any conclusions – is that celebration resists language in a way that suffering does not; or that, sometimes at least, we celebrate more by looking than speaking, by attending rather than praising. As though we sometimes celebrate when we don't know what else to do.

Another instance in the book, however, suggests something different again. The narrator has been recounting in gruesome detail the cruel history of silk manufacture and 'the great number of people', as he writes, who 'spent their lives with their wretched bodies strapped to looms made of wooden frames and rails, hung with weights, and reminiscent of instruments of torture or cages'. The work of these weavers makes it 'apparent' to him that 'we are able to maintain ourselves on this earth only by being harnessed to the machines we have invented'. And then he adds quite explicitly, in one of those Sebaldian moments when the reader isn't quite sure who the joke is on, that these weavers 'in particular' have 'much in common' with 'scholars and writers', all of whom, he writes,

> tended to suffer from melancholy and all the evils associated with it, [which] is understandable given the nature of their work, which forced them to sit bent over, day after day, straining to keep their eye on the complex patterns they created. It is difficult to imagine the depths of despair into which those can be driven who, even after the end of the working

day, are engrossed in their intricate designs and who
are pursued, into their dreams, by the feeling that
they have got hold of the wrong thread.

It is an extravagant analogy, and typically provocative. If writers and scholars are like these weavers,
then who are they being exploited by, and to what
end? Is this torturous drudgery worth the suffering?
This is a question the writers and scholars are in a
better position to consider than are the weavers. If
the lurking catastrophe is getting hold of the wrong
thread, then there must be a fantasy about the right
thread, and being able to get hold of it. What the
reader is being induced to think about are tormenting forms of authority, of lives being sacrificed and
spoiled for other people's profit.

And yet, the narrator tells us, there is something to
celebrate; the manufacturing of silk, in and of itself,
was more than merely a bad thing, even though the
entire history of silk production is an unremitting story
of tyranny. 'On the other hand,' the narrator writes,
placing us on the verge of a familiar argument,

> when we consider the weavers' mental illnesses we
> should also bear in mind that many of the materials
> produced in the factories of Norwich in the decades
> before the Industrial Revolution began – silk brocades
> and watered tabinets, satins and satinettes, camblets and
> cheveretts, prunelles, callimancoes, and florentines,

diamantines and grenadines, blondines, bombazines, belle-isles and martiniques – were of a truly fabulous variety, and of an iridescent, quite indescribable beauty as if they had been produced by Nature itself, like the plumage of birds. – That, at any rate, is what I think when I look at the marvellous strips of colour in the pattern books, the edges and gaps filled with mysterious figures and symbols.

There are in this passage stray thoughts and wrong threads; these commodities were produced by the human nature for whom Martinique was part of the slave trade. And the exotica of the list are recited with the relish of the aesthete and the knowingness of the scholar or connoisseur. When he concludes by saying, 'that, at any rate, is what I think', he is determinedly reminding us, if we needed reminding, that not everyone thinks this way about these objects, and that, earlier in the passage, neither did he.

What is being celebrated in the list of beautiful words, and the paean to variety, is the mental illness and physical torment of the people who made the objects. What would we be thinking, or indeed doing, if we were not celebrating these objects that, unlike the plumage of birds, were made by exploited labour? Is celebration a way of dehistoricizing things, a mania, a determined thoughtlessness? What are words and phrases like 'variety', 'marvellous strips of colour', or 'mysterious figures and symbols' being used

to rationalize or justify or legitimate? And of course
the narrator knows what he is doing because he pref-
aces his celebration with the most elaborate historical
account of this exploited labour, which he then com-
pares with the work of writers and scholars. Is he, as
a writer and scholar, complicit in legitimating this
suffering? In this instance, celebration, the praise and
enjoyment of beautiful, marvellous, wonderful objects,
is also a cover story. In this instance, we use our pleasure to justify the suffering of others, as if to say, if I am
enjoying these objects, or these marvellous words that
describe them, then I am not thinking about how they
are made. In this instance, celebration is a cure for
history-taking. We celebrate as a way of diverting our
attention from a history we would prefer not to know
about.

So when we celebrate books – and the narrator is
asking us to make the link – even books like Sebald's,
with what, if anything, are we being complicit? Do
we celebrate books by scholars and writers to keep
the history of how they were made – the history of
what went into their making – at bay? After the
passage I have quoted Sebald gives a characteristically
scarifying account of silk manufacture under the
Nazis, and mentions that he had come across, in
his reading, 'an old master dyer by the name of Sey-
bolt who, according to the file still in the Munich
state library was employed for nine years in a silk fac-
tory'. Silk workers are like writers and scholars; and

we are tempted sometimes to celebrate what they make in all its variety and marvellous beauty. The solution to the problem of exploitation is to celebrate what it produces, but the solution exposes the problem instead of curing it. What we are doing to objects and people when we celebrate them is one of the threads Sebald weaves into his books. Even Sebald's infamously odd photographs seem to be counter-celebratory. 'I am not seeking an answer,' he said, 'I just want to say "this is very odd indeed."'

There are, of course, two celebrations, two historically located celebrations, that haunt all of Sebald's writing, and each of them is a prelude to two different kinds of catastrophe. First, there is the celebrating of Hitler and his rise to power in Germany, and then there are the celebrations of the Allies at the end of the war. In Sebald's account, these celebrations are merely the beginning of an ongoing cultural trauma that post-war German society was unwilling or unable to acknowledge. The juxtaposition of celebration and catastrophe is integral to the kind of histories Sebald recounts, and it is done in his books more often by association than by contrivance, or, rather, by the contrivances of association that Sebald is so keen to recount. His narrators are always saying, 'this made me think of . . .' or 'this reminded me of . . .' or they are noting the free association of events called coincidences. In *Austerlitz*, for example – which reassured John Banville, writing in the *Irish Times*, that 'greatness in literature is still possible' – Austerlitz himself tells the narrator that 'only after the end of the war' could he, as a foster child from Germany, 'imagine any world outside Wales'. He knew nothing of what is referred to with appropriate understatement as 'the fighting on the continent of Europe'. 'A new epoch seemed to dawn,' he tells us, 'with the victory celebrations,' though it was also 'around the same time' that his adoptive mother Gwendolyn's 'state of health deteriorated, almost imperceptibly at first but then with increasing speed'. And it is also around this time that Austerlitz begins to know, he realizes in retrospect, about the preconditions of his own fate. He begins to realize where he has come from. The victory celebrations, and the newsreels he sees of them, are the first glimmerings he gets of his own defeatedness. And this is echoed later in the book when Vera – the neighbour who looked after him before his exile – recounts to Austerlitz how his own father, Maximilian, 'had described the Führer's prodigious reception at the Party rally' in Nuremberg:

> crowds ... stood shoulder to shoulder all agog with excitement ... the sea of radiant uplifted faces and the arms outstretched in yearning. Maximilian had told her, said Vera, that in the middle of this crowd, which had merged into a single living organism racked by strange, convulsive contractions, he

had felt like a foreign body about to be crushed and then excreted.

A few months later Austerlitz's father witnessed similar celebrations at Hitler's arrival in Vienna; 'In Maximilian's opinion ... this collective paroxysm on the part of the Viennese crowds marked the watershed.' What is referred to later in the book as 'the roars of acclamation' greeting Hitler, 'the kind of euphoria such as one feels at high altitude', are simply the prelude to horror. Whenever birthdays or Christmas are referred to, or the words 'liberation' or 'freedom' are used – and this is usually the case in all Sebald's writing – something terrible is in the offing. In Sebald's fictional documentaries, celebrations are often a sign of something else. They are always ominous, though usually only in hindsight. When Vera and Austerlitz celebrate their reunion in Prague, one of the most overwhelmingly, silently poignant moments in Sebald's writing, a terrible recounting is about to begin – about the fate of the Jews in Prague, and the Kindertransport that separated Austerlitz from his parents for ever.

If the twentieth century was, to use Eric Hobsbawm's title, *The Age of Extremes*, then it was the age of extreme celebrations. The way Sebald stages celebrations in his writing, from meetings between people to Nazi rallies, from birthdays to victory festivities, tends to make them portents of catastrophic destruction, or forms of anticipatory mourning – as though we celebrate when we are about to do terrible things or when terrible things are about to happen, as though celebrations are transitions or thresholds. But Sebald, rightly, has no truck with this kind of explicit formulation. It is, indeed, what makes his books something other than essays or theoretical writings; the many ways in which he resists being polemical contribute to what makes his books so distinctive. And yet there is a moment in his piece 'Campo Santo', one of three sections of an abandoned book about Corsica that he wrote after *The Rings of Saturn* and before *Austerlitz*, when he makes a link between celebration and mourning, and in doing so becomes suspicious.

The narrator has been talking about Corsican funeral rites, observing that they are 'extremely elaborate and of a highly dramatic character', dramatic also in the sense of sometimes seeming like 'a hollow sham, a spectacle prescribed by tradition'. But, he assures us, 'there is no discrepancy between such calculation and a genuine grief'; the 'fluctuation between the expression of deeply felt sorrow ... and the aesthetically, even cunningly modulated manipulation of the audience to whom the grief is displayed has been perhaps the most typical characteristic of our severely disturbed species at every stage of civilization'. The tentative 'perhaps' doesn't really offset the extremity of the statement, but what exactly is the nature of this disturbance? That we can make the contrived and the genuine inextricable? That authentic grief is a performance art? That we can't distinguish spontaneity from our cunning, from our wish to manipulate others? Given that mourning and, indeed, its absence, its failure in post-war Germany, are patently Sebald's themes, it is striking when these kinds of aspersions are cast – both on our own species and by implication on his own writing.

Through the idea of theatricality, Sebald then links mourning with celebration as though they were two sides of the same coin:

> Anthropological literature contains many descriptions ... of the members of early tribal cultures who, while celebrating their rites of initiation or sacrifice, retained a very precise and ever-present subliminal awareness that the compulsive extremes to which they went, always connected with the infliction of injury and mutilation, were in essence mere play-acting, even though the performance could sometimes approach the point of death. Those in severe psychological conditions also have a clear idea somewhere, in their inmost hearts, that they are literally acting body and soul in a play.

Celebration is like mourning in that they are both 'in essence mere play-acting'. It may be psychobabble, but it could still be true to say that people in severe psychological conditions know they are acting as a way of distancing themselves from the immediacy of their predicament. This still leaves us, as do Sebald's actual words, with the questions, what is the play that is being acted? and whose play is it? These questions highlight something else that obsesses Sebald about the horrifying history he did and didn't live through, and that is the complicity that sponsored it, or what the political philosopher Norma Geras has called 'the bystander phenomenon' – those who go along with terrible things by not intervening, who witness atrocities without acting. In his essay 'Constructs of Mourning', Sebald describes 'the sense of complicity and fellow-travelling that lurks hidden everywhere' in Germany. Celebration, like mourning (like writing), can have the complicity of play-acting, or so Sebald suggests. And if celebration can be a form of complicity – a form, like mourning, that conceals the fact of its complicity – we need to know what we might be complicit with in our celebrations. Writing about Peter Handke's play *Kaspar,* Sebald once suggested, in one of very few such pronouncements, that literature should keep 'faith with unsocial, banned language'. Some of the language of celebration may be too welcome, too sociable, too easy to take.

III Mendelsohn's Histories

Certain crimes are so clear
They'll never be understood.

Lawrence Raab, 'Even Clearer'

'Tell me who you desire and I will tell you your history' has become the shibboleth of post-Freudian autobiography, in which the lust for personal history has overridden the other, older kind of lust. Since everyone has a history it is now assumed that everyone has an autobiography in them. In this new solipsism we don't want other people, we want to 'recover', 'acknowledge' or 'mourn' our losses; it is not new bodies we are after but knowledge of the only past that really matters, the individual past, from which much is expected. People become interested in autobiography, Freud implies, when they lose confidence in sexuality, when sex becomes a problem, the implication being that if we could have the right kind of sexual relations then the past wouldn't bother us quite so much. Doubts about sex are doubts about the future.

This might seem a trivial account of autobiography when set against the transgenerational horror of some people's family histories, until one realizes that Freud doesn't make everything sexual, he makes everything, and particularly sexuality, a reconstruction of the past. The important thing here – and in all forms of history-writing that, like Daniel Mendelsohn's, have been affected by Freud – is not that everything is 'reduced' to sexuality, but that everything is subsumed by memory: desire for the past has all the urgency and ingenuity once accorded to sexuality. Sexuality matters because it is one's history at its most cryptically encoded. Family history shows up in one's most intimate exchanges with other people. The lost – the literal and more figurative losses from one's past – are never, in this view, quite as lost as one feared, or indeed hoped.

'Some time ago, when I was six or seven or eight years old,' Mendelsohn begins *The Lost: A Search for Six of Six Million*, 'it would occasionally happen that I'd walk into a room and certain people would begin to cry.' These people were his old Jewish relatives in Miami Beach, and they would cry because he reminded them so much of his Great-uncle Shmiel, who died in the Holocaust. 'Oh, he looks so much like Shmiel!' they would always say, as though Mendelsohn was not quite himself; as though for them he was a reminder, a living piece of family history. What was different about him was that he was strikingly similar to someone else, to one of the lost. Sameness and difference, perhaps unsurprisingly, became quite important for Mendelsohn, and so did finding out what Shmiel was really like. *The Lost* is the story of Mendelsohn's return to Bolechów, the town in Poland where Shmiel grew up and eventually died; and of Mendelsohn's recovery, as far as was possible, of what happened to Shmiel and his wife and four daughters. Who one looks like in the family is the history one has before one has a history.

One of the remarkable things about Mendelsohn's first book, *The Elusive Embrace* – which, like *The Lost*, was a kind of memoir – was the way it made connections between Mendelsohn's growing up as a gay Jewish boy in America, the son of second-generation immigrants from Eastern Europe, and his early passion for knowledge about the past, for both family history and languages. Mendelsohn is a classicist, and the whole business of knowing about and imagining lost people and cultures, of speaking unspoken languages, has been his abiding obsession. As is his sense of the difference between the propaganda of the self – our telling ourselves what we supposedly already know about ourselves – and the something else that always makes the propaganda sound ridiculous. *The Elusive Embrace* is the story of a boy who wants both to get closer and closer to his family of origin and as far away from it as possible; and in this way it is a representative story, both about the difficulties of leaving home, and the added difficulties of leaving home when the adults in the family had recently been made to leave their homes, in Mendelsohn's family's case by the Nazis. As the child of immigrants fleeing persecution one has to recover from homes having been taken away. And from languages left unused. Mendelsohn is as interested in the robbers as he is in the robbed. 'Hebrew does not really interest him,' Mendelsohn writes of himself, beginning in the third person, 'it is too close to what he already knows. Everyone he knows is Jewish; Jewish is what this flat Long Island neighbourhood is. Hebrew is not different enough. Already he has decided that he wants to learn the languages of the pagan Egyptians and Greeks and Romans, the oppressors of the ancient Hebrews.'

Since for the young Mendelsohn so-called sameness was at once taken for granted and partly rejected, and difference was the draw, his own homosexual desire was a mixed blessing. If it is difference that makes you feel alive, what is the hunger for sameness a hunger for? In *The Elusive Embrace* Mendelsohn describes homosexual desire in terms of its losses, as though what is lost or elusive for the gay man is the new, the complementary experience: gay desire is too knowing, and too knowing about the past. 'If the emotional aim of intercourse,' he writes,

> is a total *knowing* of the other, gay sex may be, in its way, perfect, because in it, a total knowledge of the other's experience is, finally, possible. But since the object of that knowledge is already wholly known

to each of the parties, the act is also, in a way, redundant. Perhaps it is for this reason that so many of us keep seeking repetition, as if depth were impossible ... when men have sex with women, they fall into the woman ... It is gay men who, during sex, fall through their partners back into themselves, over and over again.

Women are the future for a man, what Mendelsohn calls a 'destination'; the object of desire for a gay man is an unending solipsistic past, a closed circle (though it is difficult to know what 'wholly known' might mean). In this version, gay desire is a stalling of history; the gay man is driven, hopefully and hopelessly, to find the new thing, to know something other than himself. In an interesting reversal of the Freudian assumption the woman here is not so much returned to but aimed for as different, whereas gay desire is deemed to be an incessant, obsessive delving into one's personal history. Gay desire is the desire for the past, and the desire for the past that wants to pre-empt, to foreclose, the future. 'Children are the secret weapon of straight culture,' Mendelsohn writes later in the book: 'They have the potential to rescue men from inconsequentiality. Fatherhood has the power to confer authenticity on men; it can be what saves them from eternally being boys themselves.' If men need to be rescued from inconsequentiality, the future can't be that alluring for them.

What kind of history do we want, history that enables us to live in the past or history that enables us to
live in history without living in the past? History as
refuge or release, inspiration or consolation? These
were Mendelsohn's questions in *The Elusive Embrace*, a
book eloquently perplexed by a boy's appetite for
boys, a boy's appetite for family history, and a boy's
appetite for the languages of the oppressor. As Mendelsohn kept intimating, in these questions we could
read, for 'history', both history-writing and sexuality. Mendelsohn wanted to know – it is his favourite
verb in both books – what the desire for history, especially personal history, could be a desire for; and he
wanted to know what it was about the lost, the absent,
the haunting, that recruited him so effectively. *The
Lost*, like most memoirs to do with the Holocaust,
can't afford to talk too much about sexuality because
it would run the risk of trivialization, or prurience,
or complicity; but without saying so in so many words,
The Lost, like its predecessor, sees the getting of historical knowledge as akin to erotic encounter.

Mendelsohn gives as his epigraph to *The Lost* a quotation from Proust, for whom the tangle of desire and
knowledge comes out of sexual jealousy. In *The Captive*, where the quotation comes from ('When we have
passed a certain age, the soul of the child we were and
the souls of the dead from whom we have sprung
come to lavish on us their riches and their spells'),
Proust writes in excruciating detail about the way the

desire for knowledge of other people is born of exclusion. This desire is insatiable: we can never know
what we need to know about the lover because it is
not knowledge that we want but possession, a captive
to release us from our urgent burden of curiosity. For
Proust, knowledge can be the way we distract ourselves from our predicament; knowing is what we do
when there is nothing else we can do. The real torment begins when wanting turns into wanting to
know. When 'What can you know?', becomes the
question rather than 'What do you want?', sexuality
and the writing of history become daunting and obsessive. Desire becomes more violent and vengeful, and
history-writing becomes more aware of – and more
dismayed by – its necessary limitations. Knowing is
often more elusive than wanting. When wanting has
to be transformed into knowing, only the satisfactions
of narrative are available.

Once you start describing sexuality as being about
knowing people, both oneself and others, unanswer-
able questions begin to turn up. You begin to ask
yourself questions like 'Do I really know X?' rather
than 'Do I enjoy his company?' You begin to wonder
whether having a relationship with someone will be
good for you rather than whether you want to have
sex with them, and so on. Instead of taking risk and
unpredictability for granted in sexual relations, the
eradication of doubt becomes the abiding preoccupation (lovers begin to want the certainty of trust; erotic

pursuits are then more to do with safety than with shock). There is something about the quest for knowledge about other people that makes us frantic. History-writing, as Mendelsohn both shows and tells, can be a struggle to hold oneself together. Mendelsohn wrote most powerfully in *The Elusive Embrace* when he described the ways in which the boys he wanted got away from him, either through his loss of desire, or their indifference. *The Lost* tells a similar story, but the wanting is exclusively a wanting to know, and the objects of desire, so to speak, have become the six members of his family missing from the family record.

The Lost is both an attempt to reconstruct what happened to Shmiel and his family and an inquiry, more affecting because always understated, into what might make someone like Mendelsohn embark on such a gruelling quest, a quest in which the little that is known beforehand is already too much. What Mendelsohn knew of his great-uncle was his name, a few photographs, and the phrase 'killed by the Nazis'. It is the achievement of this subtle and patient book to bring this ordinary, terrible phrase back to a certain kind of life.

In Mendelsohn's account it is as if the historical imagination, like the erotic imagination, is stirred by a kind of recognition that never quite knows what it is recognizing, but can't let go of it. There is a desire to have one's desire quickened, however terrible the consequences. Mendelsohn knows that what he wants is going to horrify him. But imagining or – in his phrase – 'envisioning' his relatives' fate is the only solidarity, the only connection available to him now. There is a photograph of his great-uncle and another man, taken before the war, that Mendelsohn mentions at the beginning of *The Lost*: it is an emblem of his quest. It shows

> two young men in World War One uniforms, one of whom I knew to be the 21-year-old Shmiel while the identity of the other one was impossible to guess, unknown and unknowable ... *Unknown and unknowable*: this could be frustrating, but also produced a certain allure. The photographs of Shmiel and his family were, after all, more fascinating than the other family pictures that were so fastidiously preserved in my mother's family archive precisely because we knew almost nothing about him, about them; their unsmiling, unspeaking faces seemed, as a result, more beguiling.

Barthes reminded us that the erotic is always appearance as disappearance. If it is knowing almost nothing that is so alluring, then the quest for knowledge would seem to be about dispelling desire, relieving oneself of the burden of it. There is a certain kind of nothing, a certain kind of (elusive) object, that seems to single us out, that invites our curiosity whether we want it to or not. Mendelsohn is mindful of the fact that, in the ordinary way of things, victims of the Holocaust, and members of one's family who were victims of the Holocaust, are not supposed to be 'alluring', fascinating and beguiling. But he doesn't want to use the tragedy of the Holocaust to disguise the complicated pleasures of knowing about, or at least finding out about, the lost. It may be that we can only bear the knowledge of terrible things by getting erotic pleasure from them. These things Mendelsohn is at least willing to let us consider in his engrossing, unmelodramatic book. 'We go to tragedies,' he writes in *The Elusive Embrace*, 'because we are ashamed of our compromises, because in tragedy we find the pure beauty of absolutes.' Mendelsohn is uncompromising in *The Lost* about both the limitations and the exhilarations of his project, about the fact that it was because he was so attracted by the glamour of his great-uncle's (imagined) past that he could face discovering so exactly what the future might have held for this once successful man.

Reclaiming the story, or such facts as were available about his lost relatives, reveals to Mendelsohn just how unreclaimable they are; the more he knows, the more he knows how little his knowledge can tell him and the more he realizes that what people have to live through has few of the consolations that a story about them can offer. 'Part of my aim,' he writes, since I first began to pursue what could be known about my lost relatives, had been to try to learn whatever scraps of details about them might still be knowable, what they looked like, what their personalities were like, and yes, how they died, if anyone could still tell me that; and yet the more I talked to people, the more I was aware of how much simply can't be known, partly because the thing – the colour of her dress, the exact path she took – was never witnessed and is, therefore, unknowable now, and partly because memory itself, of those things that were witnessed, can play tricks, can elide what is too painful or be trimmed to fit a pattern that we happen to like.

What he finds himself reconstructing, essentially, the more he finds out, are the gaps in his knowledge. Knowing what he knows about these people undoes his confidence in the value of narrative coherence, of trying to get the story right. There is a difference between the (unknowably) many things that are never witnessed – both the unseen and the unnoticed – and the memories that are re-remembered for their pleasure. Even if this past could be known in the way Mendelsohn had wanted to know it, what, he keeps wondering in various ways throughout the book, would he be left with? What would it be for his quest to be successful? Once he knows as much as he knows about these people killed by the Nazis, what has he got? And if accurate reconstruction of these events is both unavailing and unavailable, what are the satisfactions being sought? *The Lost* is free of the usual facile and sentimental optimism of the those-who-are-ignorant-of-the-past-are-doomed-to-repeat-it kind. Where knowledge is not possible, acknowledgement will have to do. Mendelsohn intimates in *The Lost* that the great thing about becoming disillusioned about certain kinds of historical knowledge is that the disillusionment frees you to make certain kinds of acknowledgement. You can see what the issues are without having to overstate either the problems or their solutions.

One of the things Mendelsohn wants to acknowledge at the end of the book is that these lost relatives are not, and never were, fictional characters, even if the only life they can have now is in the memory and accounts of the living. In fact, he concludes, they may need to be rescued from the reconstructions they will now be victimized by. 'There is so much that will always be *impossible to know*,' he writes, 'but we do know that they were, once, themselves, *specific*, the subjects of their own lives and deaths, and not simply puppets to be manipulated for the purposes of a good story, for the memoirs and magical-realist novels and movies.' Like our erotic objects of desire, the one thing we resist about the dead is the reality of their lives. We have to do what we can, Mendelsohn suggests, to prevent the dead becoming objects of fantasy – as the Jews were to the Nazis – because this makes them infinitely manipulable. The most dangerous story we tell about ourselves is that people are knowable and therefore manipulable in fantasy. We should be doing whatever we can, Mendelsohn believes, to keep other people specific (that is, beyond or outside our knowledge). Whether or not they would then still be of interest to us – or, rather, what kind of interest they would have – he doesn't say. But the implication is clear: our history-writing is, by definition, non-specific, and we prefer it this way because it protects us from too much emotional impact. It is when we begin to think of the past as a manipulable object that it becomes irrecoverable. The accessible past becomes a contradiction in terms, memory as kitsch.

Visiting Auschwitz on his way to Bolechów, Mendelsohn finds the concentration camp too much of a 'symbol'. 'I thought, as I walked its strangely peaceful and manicured grounds … [that] it had been to rescue my relatives from generalities, symbols, abbreviations, to restore to them their particularity and distinctiveness, that I had come on this strange and arduous trip.' What troubled Mendelsohn in *The Elusive Embrace* about his own homosexual desire – that the particularity of the men he desired seemed to dissolve as they were endlessly replicated – becomes in *The Lost* quite explicitly a problem about the writing of history. Language, though, is a – if not *the* – medium of repetition, so there is a sense in which Mendelsohn is asking of language something that it cannot do. Language and memory, and language as memory, necessarily set limits to particularity, and these limits protect us from what we would rather not feel or imagine. Mendelsohn wants the kind of particularity that writing, however good, can never give; language estranges us from an immediacy we may not be able to bear. Indeed, we might ask of any object we value – a language, a book, a person, a moral ideal – what does it help us to forget? Rescuing one's relatives from generalities, symbols and abbreviations – if it were possible – would be more than most people could take, though acknowledging that may be of use. We suffer most, Mendelsohn sometimes intimates, from the ways we have of avoiding our suffering. He wants his history-writing to be a way of talking about this.

The Lost continually plays off historical fact against individual memory, academic research against felt experience. This is not a new thing to do, but Mendelsohn does it with unusual perspicacity. He discovered in the *Holocaust Encyclopedia*, for example, that in the first mass liquidation of the Jews in Bolechów some were 'tortured for 24 hours'. He asked a very old lady in Bolechów what

'being tortured for 24 hours' might mean. She told us that the Jews had been herded into the Catholic community centre at the northern edge of the town, and that there the Germans had forced the captive Jews to stand on each other's shoulders, and had placed the old rabbi on the top; then knocked him down. Apparently this went on for many hours.

Generalities, symbols and abbreviations can be horrifying enough; the stories, in detail, Mendelsohn finds virtually unbearable. Hundreds of Jews were shot in mass graves, as everyone knew, but one of the surviving villagers told Mendelsohn that 'the earth continued to move for days after the shootings, because not all of the victims were actually dead when the grave was filled in'. The noise of the gunfire was so terrible that the old lady's mother, as they sat in their house, 'took down a decrepit old sewing machine and ran the treadle, so that the creaky noise would cover the gunfire'. The closer he gets to the lived experience of these events, the more intimate they become, the more intimacy – in its various senses – becomes Mendelsohn's subject. Our prizing of closeness – both our intimacies with others, and the sympathetic intimacies created by certain kinds of historical writing – may be an addiction to hatred or fear, or to both. What makes us think, or why would we want to think, that the more we know about people the more we will like them? 'It is a matter of recorded fact,' Mendelsohn writes, 'that many of the most violent savageries carried out against the

Jews of Eastern Europe were perpetrated not by the Germans themselves, but by the local populations ... the neighbours, the intimates, with whom the Jews had lived side by side for centuries.' Many people find this incomprehensible, or, as Mendelsohn puts it, 'strange – not least the Jews themselves'.

But, as Mendelsohn points out, family members, everybody's first intimates, are usually something of a problem: 'Being so intimate,' he writes, 'having too much access to what goes on inside those closest to you by blood ... will sometimes have an opposite reaction, causing family members to flee one another, to seek more – we use the literal and figurative terms interchangeably, these days – "space".' Our history-writing can be our phobia of the past. Interspersing the account of his journey with biblical commentary, most notably on the Cain and Abel story, Mendelsohn makes a sober case for the savagery of family life. It is a seemingly obvious point, but apparently an easy one to forget, that family members have the strongest of mixed – or even opposing – feelings about one another. This may tell us less about human nature than about the dangers of assuming human relations have something to do with knowing oneself and others. When knowing is what you spend your time doing, this is what you get, the need for more 'space', *Lebensraum*. If you get too close to the historical record you begin to think of closeness as both the problem and the point.

Along the way, as Mendelsohn travels to a great many countries and meets many remarkable people – the book is packed with extraordinary encounters between people with a shared history that they are more or less able or willing to acknowledge – he tries to formulate this issue of distance, where the personal and the historical overlap. For Mendelsohn it is not so much about getting the distance right as conceding that the regulation of distance is what is at issue. 'Proximity,' he ventures at one point, 'brings you closer to what happened, is responsible for the facts we glean, the artefacts we possess, the verbatim quotations of what people said; but distance is what makes possible the story of what happened, is precisely what gives someone the freedom to organize and shape those bits into a pleasing and coherent whole.' This is the conventional view, and indeed the way many men think of their lives: you get the best version when you get away. What makes *The Lost* unconventional is the way Mendelsohn comes to suspect that this very freedom to organize and shape is complicit with so many of the things he fears most: the tyrannies of exclusion, the manipulation of material. However well drawn the characters, however good the story, we are always aware of what has been lost in the making.

IV Auden's Magic

> What is heartening about people is their appalling
> stubbornness and the strong roots of their various
> cultures, rather than the ease with which you can
> convert them and make them happy and good.

> William Empson, review of Auden's *Another Time* in
> *Life & Letters Today*, August 1940

Reviewing T. S. Eliot's *A Choice of Kipling's Verse* in the *New Republic* in 1943 Auden made a series of distinctions that were to reverberate through his later work. 'Art, as the late Professor R. G. Collingwood pointed out,' Auden points out:

> is not Magic, i.e., a means by which the artist communicates or arouses his feelings in others, but a mirror in which they may become conscious of what their own feelings really are: its proper effect, in fact, is disenchanting.
>
> By significant details it shows us that our present state is neither as virtuous nor as secure as we thought, and by the lucid pattern into which it unifies these details, its assertion that order is possible, it faces us with the command to make it actual. Insofar as he is an artist, no one, not even Kipling, is intentionally a

magician. On the other hand, no artist, not even Eliot, can prevent his work being used as magic, for that is what all of us, highbrow and lowbrow alike, secretly want Art to be.

This account is informed by the young Auden's Freudianism; the Freudian analyst – in the same way as what Auden calls Art – does not deliberately arouse or communicate his feelings in the others who are his patients but offers them, in Freud's own analogy, a mirror 'in which they may become conscious of what their own feelings really are'. It is easy to see how the psychoanalyst might do this, or attempt to, but more difficult to see how a poem would. The Freudian analyst, for example, does it by a calculated reticence and an unforthcoming manner; he speaks only to enable the patient to hear himself. In what sense, then, can poems be like Freudian analysts? And why, not to mention how, should they aspire to be so? The answer to the 'why' question is that Auden, writing here in 1943, wants Art to be the articulation of what Freud called the Reality Principle, and which Auden refers to as disenchantment; that is, a consciousness of what one's feelings really are. For Auden, at this time – to put it in the kind of schematic way the young Auden was drawn to in his prose – there was Art and there was Religion and there was Politics, and between them there was Magic as the temptation that threatened to corrupt them, that distracted people from

what they really felt. Was it possible, Auden was asking, for Art, or poetry – his chosen art – not to be
wishful? What can one believe about words if one
doesn't believe that they are magic?

Having recognized, as one might in a Freudian
analysis, and, indeed, during a world war, that, as
Auden writes, 'our present state is neither as virtuous
nor as secure as we thought', we are faced with what
Auden calls the 'command' to make the 'lucid pattern'
– the 'order' that is art – actual. Art is one of the ways
we have of perceiving the true order – what we really
feel, the way things really are – and of abiding by it.
So no artist would intentionally be a magician because
no artist would seek to mislead, to lie to his audience; and, more troublingly, no artist can prevent his
work being used as magic – as wishfully consoling, as
distractingly entertaining, as wilfully seductive –
because, as Auden puts it in his ominously knowing
way – which he calls in a poem 'the preacher's loose
immodest tone' – 'that is what all of us, highbrow
and lowbrow alike, secretly want Art to be'. Secretly,
presumably because we know we shouldn't, because
Art as Magic is a forbidden and illegitimate pleasure,
and because what we are ashamed of wanting most
are our wishful apprehensions. The big secret about
Art is that no one wants it to be true. Apart, that is,
from the artist, who we might think Auden has a little
wishfully exempted – no artist 'is intentionally a
magician' – while telling us that lowbrows and high-

brows alike want art to be magic, and, presumably, the artist is prone to be unintentionally a magician. The audience can't resist the allure of magic, so how can the artist? What was enchanting about Auden, his magic, was exactly what he came to distrust. Art must disenchant without making disenchantment itself enchanting.

'My parents were Anglo-Catholics,' Auden wrote in 1934, 'so that my first religious memories are of exciting magical rites ... rather than of listening to sermons.' Auden's early poetry is a mixture of exciting magical rites – both verbal and formal – and sermonizing; but if you begin to distrust the magic – indeed, see the function of art as dispelling the magic, as disillusionment – what, if any, is the alternative to sermonizing? Once you abjure magic do you have to become preachy, or dogmatic, or amusingly dull, or just knowingly frivolous? (In Barbara Everett's words, once Auden renounced 'that eager desire to convince at least himself of the permanent value of an idea', he was 'transmuted into the soberer, barely perceptible dogmatism of the visiting professor, whose most militant postulate is entrenched in a polite epigram'.) Auden could not give up on the eager desire to convince at least himself of the harm that magic does.

Magic is dangerous, for Auden, because it involves the pretence that one can live outside the law, of both Man and God (it is literally antisocial because it is a form of inattention). It is a corrupt form of specialness.

In *The Prolific and the Devourer*, a book of aphorisms and reflections begun and abandoned in 1939, Auden wrote of the sin of idolatry that 'an idol is someone or something that one believes to be above the law. And to worship one, whether a person, or institution, or dogma is to abandon Faith for belief, Science for magic.' For Auden in 1939 there is Science and Faith, with capital letters, and lower-case belief and magic. In the name of Truth, Art must be the enemy of credulity. Sermonizing again much later in 1963 in the Postscript to *The Dyer's Hand* Auden draws his consistent thread – which in *The Sea and the Mirror*, written in 1942–4, was being worked out, and had not hardened into an attitude – about magic as disingenuous, and about what the alternatives to it might be. This, indeed, is the consistent thread; Auden seeing magic as the thing to which we must find an alternative; magic as both threat and promise, the thing about which he must protest too much, that he must insist on warning us against. 'Man desires to be free and he desires to feel important,' Auden writes in *The Dyer's Hand*:

This places him in a dilemma, for the more he emancipates himself from necessity the less important he feels.

That is why so many actes gratuites are criminal: a man asserts his freedom by disobeying a law and retains a sense of self-importance because the law he has disobeyed is an important one. Much crime is magic, an attempt to make free with necessity.

An alternative to criminal magic is the innocent game. Games are actes gratuites in which the players obey rules chosen by themselves. Games are freer than crimes because the rules of a game are arbitrary and moral laws are not; but they are less important.

One possible schema would be something like: Auden began by being intrigued by, if not believing in, magic; then he soon realized that magic was the problem not the solution, and that Art could be the necessary and useful enemy of magic, exposing its depredations of the soul. Then Religion, the Christian communion that Auden returned to in 1940, became the self-cure for magic; and then Art became an alternative – a kind of compromise-formation, to use Freud's language – to magic, because it was not strong enough to wholeheartedly resist the blandishments of magic, was indeed keen to incorporate a bit of magic in its truthfulness, but was, at best, trading with the enemy, not, at worst, capitulating. Art in short became what Auden calls here an act gratuit, the innocent game that is an alternative to criminal magic because instead of breaking the rules of Authoritative Others the players of the innocent game of art 'obey rules chosen by themselves'. Where once evasive harm was committed now there is gratuitous and satisfying minor accomplishment. Art is put in its place by exposing magic.

In his 1952 lectures on Auden, Randall Jarrell has this to say about Auden's *The Age of Anxiety*, the volume of poems published in 1948, after *The Sea and the Mirror*:

> One understands what Auden meant when he said, in a recent review, that all art is so essentially frivolous that he prefers it to embody beliefs he thinks false, since its frivolity would degrade those he thinks true. This sounds like an indictment of art, but it is also a confession of Auden's, and *The Age of Anxiety* is the evidence that substantiates the confession. It is the sort of poem that an almost absolutely witty, and almost absolutely despairing, dictionary would write.

Whether or not one agrees with Jarrell – and there is the kind of bitter disillusionment in these words that suggests a great hope betrayed – there is, as it were, a sea-change being worked out in *The Sea and the Mirror*. *The Age of Anxiety* is a quite different kind of poem. 'Underneath the jokes and fantasies and sermons,' Jarrell continues, 'there is a chaotic, exhausted confusion ... (During the late 1940s [that is, after *The Sea and the Mirror*] Auden's poetry, which had been under extraordinary moral, political and theological tension for many years, now and then collapsed into the most abject frivolity)'. The Postscript in *The Dyer's Hand* was subtitled 'The Frivolous and the Earnest'; if poetry couldn't ultimately counter, or countermand, magic it could, at least, be a

pleasurable game. 'Underneath the jokes and fantasies
and sermons' and commentary and polemic and
astounding virtuosity and verbal intelligence of *The
Sea and the Mirror* there is not a 'chaotic, exhausted
confusion', but an inspired engagement with, among
other things, the place of magic in art. Here we find
above all both the performance of, and the inquiry
into, what Seamus Heaney has called Auden's 'con-
stant return' to 'the double nature of poetry'; and it
is magic that Heaney has to talk about. 'On the one
hand,' he writes, in *The Government of the Tongue*, for
Auden,

> poetry could be regarded as magical incantation, fun-
> damentally a matter of sound and the power of sound
> to bind our minds' and bodies' apprehensions within an
> acoustic complex; on the other hand, poetry is a matter
> of making wise and true meanings, of commanding
> our emotional assent by the intelligent disposition
> and inquisition of human experience. In fact most
> poems – including Auden's – constitute temporary
> stays against the confusion threatened by the mind's
> inclination to accept both accounts of poetic function in
> spite of their potential mutual exclusiveness. But 'con-
> fusion' is probably far too strong a word, since Auden is
> able to make a resolving parable of the duality, assigning
> the beauty/magic part to Ariel and the truth/meaning
> part to Prospero and proposing that every poem, indeed
> every poet, embodies a dialogue between them.

Heaney is using *The Sea and the Mirror* here to create resolution – 'a resolving parable' – where resolution may be neither possible nor the point. (He noticeably draws back from the blessings of confusion.) Magic is invoked in different registers – there is the magic of incantation, the suasive power of the sound of words, and the magic as embodied, so to speak, in Ariel's words – but *The Sea and the Mirror* also proffers an alternative to mutual exclusiveness or dialogue or resolving parables of duality. Magic in the poem can be neither excluded nor included; so the 'confusion' that Heaney thinks is too strong a word in Auden's case, and which Jarrell diagnosed in *The Age of Anxiety*, is germane to the ethos of the poem. Confusion – the fog that holds contradictions together – is often what Auden's best poetry is staving off, and trying to think about: because one of the things that magic does is confuse; it shows us something about the nature of confusion. It confuses our sense of reality by showing us an alternative reality, always a contradiction in terms. Magic lets confusion into the poem. Another way of saying this is what Auden wrote to Stephen Spender about the 'subject' of *The Sea and the Mirror*: 'the serious matter being the fundamental frivolity of art'. Auden wants to consign magic to the 'frivolity of art'. As we begin to consider *The Sea and the Mirror* we should bear in mind Christopher Isherwood's note of 1936: 'Auden loathed (and still rather dislikes) the sea – for the sea,

besides being deplorably wet and sloppy, is formless.'
If confusion is the enemy of form, and formlessness
is deplorable, then choice of form and forms of choice
become paramount considerations.

In his 1949 lectures at the University of Virginia
on *The Enchafèd Flood* Auden didn't have a good word
for the sea. 'The sea or the great waters,' he writes,

> are the symbol for the primordial undifferentiated
> flux, the substance which became created nature
> only by having form imposed or wedded to it.
>
> The sea, in fact, is that state of barbaric vagueness
> and disorder out of which civilisation has emerged
> and into which, unless saved by the efforts of gods and
> men, it is always liable to relapse. It is so little of a
> friendly symbol ... The sea is no place to be if you can
> help it, and to try to cross it betrays a rashness border-
> ing on hubris, at which a man's friends should be
> properly concerned.

The sea, like Art, is disenchanting, but unlike Art
it is 'undifferentiated flux'. Again the issue is about
form; art unifying the details into a 'lucid pattern'
reveals, in the words of Eliot's Kipling review, 'that
order is possible [and] actual'. The sea, for Auden, as
Isherwood noted, 'is formless', the mirror shows
us, gives us back, the actuality of form. Magic, we
infer, isn't formlessness but bad form. Magic, unlike
a mirror, imposes an impossible, an unreal, order; the

sea needs to have 'form imposed upon or wedded to it'. In reading *The Sea and the Mirror* we need to bear in mind the difference between an imposition and a wedding, and the kinds of form proposed and imposed by gods and men for 'the primordial undifferentiated flux' that gods and men are up against. Mirrors are good, in Auden's poetic universe; magic and the sea are not. They are, in fact, a mortal danger; false order and no order. Mirrors are, in their traditional role, only able to show us what is there to be seen (but in reflection, a rather important difference; mirrors do not show us what is there, but what is reflected). Like all of Auden's many schemas, it is the confusion felt rather than the order imposed that is the most striking.

The way Auden and later commentators have talked about *The Sea and the Mirror* make it sound rather programmatic, a work of art with a project: an attempt to sort something out. It has been noted, for example, that in June 1942 Auden wrote in a letter to Ursula Niebuhr that *The Sea and the Mirror* 'is really about the Christian conception of art'; and Auden followed this up with an article in *The Commonweal* in November of the same year in which he wrote: 'As a writer, who is also a would-be Christian, I cannot help feeling that a satisfactory theory of art from the standpoint of Christian faith has yet to be worked out.' Clearly in his own mind *The Sea and the Mirror* has an animating intention, constituting, in Arthur Kirsch's words, 'Auden's attempt, with

the example of *The Tempest*, to work out that theory'
of art from the standpoint of Christian faith. But
there is a risk, in reading the poem, that in seeing the
resolutions sought (and perhaps achieved) one under-
rates the conflicts and confusions contended with.
That we might, as Auden wants us to, prefer the
solution, such as it is, to the problems that prompted
it. We need to bear in mind, I think, Jarrell's words
that after *The Sea and the Mirror*, 'Auden's poetry,
which had been under extraordinary moral, political
and theological tension for many years, now and
then collapsed into the most abject frivolity.' The
dismissal is excessive, as I said, because the disillusionment was so great; but it may be the 'extraordinary moral, political and theological tension' of
The Sea and the Mirror that matters most. That even if
the poem is, in John Fuller's words, Auden's 'self-
confessed ars poetica', we should not assume that
the 'theory of art from the standpoint of Christian
faith' had been worked out, or worked out successfully, in the poem. Indeed, the poem might succeed
because the project failed; that his attempt to work
out a Christian conception of art diminished art by
revealing its essential frivolity in the scheme of
things, and yet if a poem could do this it could not,
itself, be frivolous. Jarrell, of course, intimates that
Auden wasn't seeking a Christian conception of art
but release from the 'extraordinary moral, political
and theological tension' that had constituted his

poetic vocation. As though Christianity freed Auden from taking art too seriously; the vocation of becoming a Christian as a refuge from the vocation of being a poet. *The Sea and the Mirror* then becomes many things: an elegy for Auden's ambitions as a poet, and for poetry (and for art as magic: the poet who needs to write that poetry makes nothing happen may once have believed that it could make anything or everything happen); a poem about the perils of seeking resolution where resolution may not be possible; a poem about the terrors of confusion, of chaos, of formlessness. It is worth seeing, in other words, what the poem sounds like if we don't put our faith, as Auden did, in the Christianity, but in the poetry; if we read the poem for its extraordinary tensions rather than what Barbara Everett called its 'central lyrical vision of harmony'. Of *The Sea and the Mirror* she writes: 'By brilliant technical means ... Auden comes very near to achieving perfectly his end; to show the fusion of all dualities, of Art and Life, of individual and community, and of the warring desires of the mind.' It is, I think, a better poem about the difficulties of sustaining conflict, about what is at stake in confusion, about how hard it is to keep one's balance, as the very first lines of the poem suggest:

> The aged catch their breath,
> For the nonchalant couple go
> Waltzing across the tightrope

As if there were no death
Or hope of falling down.

Led by these opening lines I want to briefly show
Auden also showing us just how misleading, how
distracting, the desire for resolution is. The settling
of the unsettlable. We can also, the poem suggests, be
paid on both sides and keep our balance, 'straddling
the conflicts', in Empson's words. Magic is what we
use as the antidote to this, and we need to see what
the word is doing in the poem. If Christianity isn't
magic, and Art mustn't be magic – though there is
usually some magic about it in Auden's view – what
has magic got that Auden doesn't want?

On the few occasions Auden uses the word 'magic'
or refers to it in *The Sea and the Mirror* he seems to
use it to remind us of the conflicts, the tensions, that
would have to be borne without it. And they are
tensions, that do not always admit of plausible resolution, Christian or otherwise. Auden tells us in
some detail early in Chapter One of the poem what
magic was a solution to for Prospero; at this point in
the poem Auden clearly wants us to take the problem seriously, and Prospero's problem, in Auden's
account, is the ordinary problem of growing up:

When I woke into my life, a sobbing dwarf
Whom giants served only as they pleased, I was not
    what I seemed;

Beyond their busy backs I made a magic
To ride away from a fathers imperfect justice,
    Take vengeance on the Romans for their grammar,
Usurp the popular earth and blot out for ever
    The gross insult of being a mere one among many;
Now Ariel, I am that I am, your late and lonely master,
    Who knows now what magic is; – the power to enchant
That comes from disillusion.

Magic, at least for the child, dispels the experience of
the nothing that comes from not being all. Prospero
escapes 'a fathers imperfect justice', the tyranny of
grammar, and the insult of being 'a mere one among
many'. Magic is defined in one of Auden's compelling formulations as: 'the power to enchant/ That
comes from disillusion'. The implication being that
there is something about disillusionment – or about
certain disillusionments – that cannot be borne.
Given every child, and therefore every adult, experiences these disillusionments, Auden through Prospero makes us wonder what would be a better coming
to terms, what would be better terms, to meet such
formative, such constitutive human experiences? There
is, of course, a glimmer of hope in the implication
that one would not need to ride away from a father's
imperfect justice if one had God for a father, whose
justice is by definition perfect; and one's insignificance
might be redeemed by being loved by God; but grammar, the poets' medium, would remain the same.

What would happen, we are invited to wonder, if the disillusionments were acknowledged without the saving grace of Christianity, or the cover-up of magic? It is Antonio, the usurping brother, who speaks up most forcefully for our inability to take our disillusionments seriously; that is, seriously enough to abjure magic. For Antonio there is something ineluctable about Prospero's magic:

> Break your wand in half
> The fragments will join; burn your books or lose
> Them in the sea, they will soon reappear,
> Not even damaged: as long as I choose
>
> To wear my fashion, whatever you wear
> Is a magic robe; while I stand outside
> Your circle, the will to charm is still there.

The threat of usurpation – of being replaced or made to submit – makes magic essential; as long as an Antonio figure lurks – as long as he chooses to wear his fashion, to stand outside – magic, as if by magic, will reconstitute itself as the best defence born of terror. Faced with the Evil that Auden tends to capitalize – and reinforced by news from the war – there is recourse to the magic that sustains magic; broken wands mend themselves, burnt and lost books reappear. 'The will to charm is still there'; and that is also, of course, Will Shakespeare. We have the magic of art that we may not perish of the truth.

By 1947, in his lecture on *The Tempest* at the New
School, New York, Auden is still keen to expose
Prospero's magic, but for more pragmatic reasons; it
is not so much an Evil – a hubristic usurping of God,
an inability to bear the disillusion of being human –
but an ineffectual thing. It doesn't do enough. 'What
can't magic do?' Auden asks apropos of Prospero
abjuring his: 'It can give people an experience, but
it cannot dictate the use they make of that experience ... That art cannot transform men grieves Prospero greatly. His anger at Caliban stems from his
consciousness of this failure ... You can hold a mirror up to a person but you may make him worse.'
The terms have shifted: art as magic can be a mirror
but mirrors can make people worse; magic gives an
experience but cannot determine or predict what
will be done with it, what 'use', to use Auden's pragmatic American word, it will be put to. Art, like
Shakespeare's, might be the very best thing people are
capable of, but it is insufficient. The best things about
people are not good enough. Human nature, without
divine redemption, is a disillusionment that cannot
be borne. Charm, enchantment, books, wands, robes,
magic, mirrors, even art itself; they are all insufficient.
But art, like *The Tempest*, like *The Sea and the Mirror*,
can at least show us why art is never fully adequate,
what believing in art as magic deprives us of. Something had become unbearable to Auden and he wanted
to call it human nature, unredeemed human nature.

As an epigraph to his *Collected Poems* of 1976, dedi-
cated to Christopher Isherwood and Chester Kall-
man, Auden wrote:

> Although you be, as I am, one of those
> Who feel a Christian ought to write in prose,
> For poetry is magic: born in sin, you
> May read it to exorcise the Gentile in you.

Auden opens his *Collected Poems* with a definition of
what poetry is: 'poetry is magic', and with an account
of what this particular magic may be for: 'to exorcise
the Gentile in you' (Fuller helpfully glosses 'Gentile'
as 'Heathen'; 'gentile' originally meaning, like 'Heathen', neither a gentile nor a Jew). Could Auden possibly mean that poetry is the magic that might prepare
you for the true faith, or is this some kind of joke? At
the very end, and at the very beginning of his *Collected
Poems*, Auden couldn't or didn't want to separate out
his magic from his poetry.

Mothers and Fairy Tales

'I hate subtleties,' said Ursula ... 'I always
think they are a sign of weakness.'

D. H. Lawrence, *The First 'Women in Love'*

I Jack and His Beanstalk

A story is told of Alfred Adler, one of Freud's early fol-
lowers, who once interviewed a prospective patient at
great length, taking a detailed family history, and getting as elaborate an account as possible of what the man
was suffering from. At the end of this three-hour con-
sultation Adler apparently said to the man, 'What
would you do if you were cured?' The man answered
him, and Adler said, 'Well, go and do it then.' That was
the treatment. As in 'Jack and the Beanstalk', as in many
fairy stories, there is a serious problem, and a piece of
magic; and the magic makes strange things possible.
What the magic is there to do is to show us just how
poor our sense of possibility always is. Jack's beans make
him full of beans; they make his world huge. And show
him, of course, as a foretaste of big things to come – that

is, his living happily ever after with his beautiful princess after the end of the end of his story – that very small things can get bigger and lead you into unexpected and unusually satisfying places. Small boys are not Freudians but they know they have their own beanstalk; and that it takes them away from life at home.

What Adler's interpretation, like a lot of psychoanalytic interpretation, suggested was that this man was suffering from missed opportunities, from uncompleted actions. As though, Adler was intimating, people suffer from not having been able to take their chances; that for reasons of which they were unconscious they couldn't use what happened to them for the satisfactions they were seeking. They couldn't, as Jack certainly can, make their wishes come true enough. Jack saves his mother and himself from destitution (and pleasing himself pleases his mother, always a bit of an issue in ordinary life), gets an adventure and gets the gold, outwits and kills the child-eating giant, makes himself and his mother very rich, marries a beautiful princess and lives happily ever after. Unlike real life, in which you can solve a problem only by creating another one, Jack solves all his problems, and the solution gives him a conflict-free life.

Adler's patient needed to be reminded of what he actually did want to do, and to get a picture of the risks involved, of what the catastrophes were, both real and imagined, that were inhibiting him. Jack, of course, only needs magic beans to get what he wants, to carry out his desires; so the story shows us that you need something called luck, but luck does happen, and you can make something out of your luck. On his way to selling the cow Jack meets a stranger – who oddly knows his name, so the world is somehow working for Jack – who gives him the magic beans in exchange for the cow. From his mother's point of view he has made a terrible mistake, but the tale reassures us all – and particularly children – that mistakes can work, that naivety makes extraordinary things possible whereas worldliness, the making of good deals, can secure your survival, but not grant you undreamed-of success. The story says, being sensible only gets you sensible things. And whatever else childhood is it is an initiation into the sensible.

The child, in other words, is learning what is to be done; and Freud added to our picture of what can be done in the child's mind that can and can't be done in the so-called shared world. Desires occur to us as wishes, and wishes occur to children as being possible actions. Some actions, from the adult's point of view, are clearly uncompletable – the little boy doesn't have the wherewithal to marry his mother, which for Jack translates as his being unable to earn a living and 'support' her – and have to be acknowledged as such. Some actions are or seem to be too dangerous to complete – the boy trying to kill his sibling: one of the satisfying things about Jack's story is that there are no siblings, and no couples with children, so Jack has no rivals and is irredeemably special – and have to be shied away from. And with some wishes it's just not obvious what completion would be: the child doesn't always know whether the meal is finished when he has eaten everything on his plate, or when he is full, or when he has just had enough (Jack solves this 'magically' by knowing and getting exactly what he wants, and in its satisfying him for ever). It is in childhood that these essential perplexities, which never end, which live happily (and unhappily) ever after, begin. And, unsurprisingly perhaps, fairy stories are full of them. They are about what children like Jack can and can't do with their wishes; about what happens, and what might happen, if you do what you seem to want to do.

So it isn't that fairy tales, or indeed children, are Freudian but that Freud's insights are childish (in the best sense) and fairy-tale like. What psychoanalysis adds to the conversation is the wish to make sexuality explicit. The psychoanalyst assumes that the so-called patient is unaware of the actions he wants to complete, of the opportunities he has missed. And that what he desires, and the ways in which he desires it, has been made unconscious out of fear (all fairy tales are studies in fear). The trouble is that when the militant psychoanalyst interprets fairy tales we usually end up with a list of the forbidden or unacceptable desires that the story has managed more or less artfully to disguise. As though the fairy story – however frightening or gruesome – is the good-manners

version and the psychoanalytic interpretation is the
bad-manners version. What has been revealed, supposedly, is why the child, unbeknown to himself,
likes the story: because it enacts, it dramatizes, his
most enticing and forbidden wishes in a pleasurable
way, that is, it is amusing and exciting. But no one
who likes reading, or pantomimes, could possibly like
reading these translations because they try to make
the commentary, the interpretation, sound more convincing than the story itself. There are good reasons
why knowing about the Oedipus complex never
replaces seeing or reading *Hamlet*. The story goes on
working because it can't be explained away. So the
question is: what, if anything, has a psychoanalytic
interpretation got to add to this? Not, what is the
story really about, but what does it make you go on
thinking about, or wanting to say? 'Jack and the
Beanstalk' clearly says something, as story and as pantomime, to children, and therefore must say something about children (and, of course, about the adults
who want them to experience it). It must say something about their fascinations and misgivings about
growing up; about what it is, as a child, to take your
chances, as Jack does when he grasps an opportunity
where there doesn't seem to be one. Fairy stories are
a way children can consider their options.

The most striking thing, from a psychoanalytic
point of view, is how the story begins. The they-
lived-happily-ever-after ending is a way of saying

there are no more stories in this story; the story of desire and its obstacles can come to an end. Whereas the beginning of 'Jack and the Beanstalk' is a perennial human predicament, one of the sources of all conflict, the moment when a mother and a child realize their insufficiency as a unit, echoed in adulthood when lovers discover that they can't be everything for each other, and they need something or somebody else. Jack and his mother, a 'poor widower', are dependent on their cow – rather too literally, too psychoanalytically, called Milky-white – who one day gives no milk, and so they have to sell her. It is, alas, a weaning story; and weaning stories involve a quest for new resources, and the freedom of having new, more various needs. When weaning works it opens up the world. And the story reassures everyone involved, particularly the spectators, because once Milky-white has been traded for the magic beans, things get better and better for Jack and his mother – that is to say, they become exorbitantly wealthy and Jack, at least, finds the princess of his dreams (what happens to his mother, needless to say, is dropped as an issue; mothers are people who have no future). On the way to getting rid of Milky-white, getting rid of their need for her, Jack discovers that strange men are the answer, the strangeness of men – the magic beans they possess, their desire to eat children and bully women (that is, not be bullied by them) – presumably being the strangeness he will acquire in growing up. The women in the story are either miserable and bad-tempered (Jack's mother) or protective and helpful and placating of men (the giant's wife); but the covert, cheery message in the story is that mother and son are both better off if the son is dependent on the mother rather than vice versa. Indeed, that growing up is a process of turning the tables: the mother supports the son, then the son supports the mother. Weaning is the process in which the child makes the mother dependent on him, while leaving her for another woman. Some children might find this an exhilarating prospect, but few mothers would. All the good things in the story, it should be noted, come from the men, magic beans and gold.

So if, as in the story, mothers either let you down or help you outwit their monstrous husbands when they are not procuring and cooking children for these husbands to eat, what do fathers do? If the mothers 'use' Jack, to make money or harm their husbands, what do the fathers in the story want? Jack, after all, as a boy is in some sense like them. The first man who mysteriously gives Jack the magic beans is in some enigmatic way inordinately helpful, even though Jack doesn't understand why the man is willing to trade the cow for the beans, and Jack's mother is furious and throws the beans away. This man, though not recognized as a good man, saves their lives and makes their fortune. So the story says rather straightforwardly but rather puzzlingly at the same time, as is the way with fairy tales, a good man – whose goodness will be unintelligible, will look like a trick and will require faith – and some good luck are all you need (Jack was lucky enough to bump into the man with the beans, and when his mother threw the beans away in a rage they luckily landed somewhere they could grow). A woman, one way or another, will want something from you; a man will want something for you (the beans man seems utterly altruistic). But there is another kind of man – the other side of being a man, as it were – who lives on children and enslaves women; who, because he eats children, wants everything from children, their lives (the women in the story, other than Jack's future princess, may be exploitative, but they are not killers, they are not the ultimate kind of parasite). And it is this one that poses the most interesting problem for Jack: with the beans man, Jack simply had to accept, on trust, the beans; accept that he was dealing with a man of his word; with the giant (or ogre, as he is called in some versions) Jack has to steal his wealth, his potency, but without becoming like him.

If we say for the sake of argument that the giant represents a potential version of Jack's future self, then Jack has to find a way of becoming potent without becoming brutal. The first stage of potency is accepting on trust that there is such a thing as magic power (for the child an erection is magic); the second stage is being ingenious enough to be potent without having to be too cruel. Of course, as in all fairy stories, there are enigmatic implications everywhere: Jack makes his fortune and his future from the giant's gold – the gold coins, the hen that lays the golden egg, the golden harp – but how did the giant get it? All money is dirty money; all potency is dirty potency. When Jack has to kill the giant in order to save his own life, he is allowed to because it has become expedient, so Jack doesn't have to feel quite so guilty; he hadn't set out to kill the giant, he had just set out to get his gold. At least that's the story Jack can tell himself. Jack, it would seem, has got nothing to feel too bad about, and he has succeeded beyond his wildest dreams.

But perhaps, above all, Jack's real triumph – a triumph that would surely appeal to everyone watching the pantomime – is that Jack has pleased himself by pleasing his mother. By fulfilling his mother's wishes he has fulfilled his own. Jack seems to have been able to provide her with exactly what she needs; the abject, poverty-stricken widower is transformed by his daring into a happy woman: 'Jack and his mother became very rich,' the story ends, 'and he married a great princess, and they lived happily ever after.' '[T]hey', though ambiguous, could mean all of them. The mother didn't have another child, and she didn't have another man; as it turned out, her son was all she needed. If money is all anyone really needs then no one has to grow up. Jack is the boy who succeeds by never letting his mother down. Jack, in other words, is the boy who can't bear being hated by his mother, who will become the man who never grows up because he can't bear being hated by a woman; unlike the giant, who can only be hated by a woman, who has to keep doing terrible things to a woman to show himself that he can survive her hatred. Or Jack might become a man who keeps finding magic beans, who can be potent without doing harm. But the story ends with Jack nicely set up for a perfect future. The boy he was has made him the man he will be. Like the crudest of Freudians the story implies that for Jack all the significant things have happened in his childhood. If Jack ever wants to understand his own life all he will have to do is see (or read) 'Jack and the Beanstalk'.

II The Least of Her Problems:
Cinderella and Men

Freud's infamous question 'What does a woman want?' is both silly and mildly insulting, implying as it does that women in general are incapable of knowing what their wants are and making them known; aside from the obvious fact that all women are different and want different things at different times. What Freud really wanted to know, by asking this question, is what do mothers want from their children? It is a question all of us, as children (and not only as children), are endlessly exercised by: what did our mothers want us for?

Cinderella is a girl with three mothers: a mother who has died (about whom we know nothing); a wicked stepmother; and a fairy godmother. And this translates as: a mysterious mother whose wishes are unknown; a mother who hates and sabotages Cinderella's pleasure; and a mother who does everything she can to support it. So the story suggests, among other things, that there is something strangely magical, at least from the girl's point of view, about the mother who is devoted to her daughter's pleasure (as opposed to being devoted to her daughter). Like all the best fairy stories 'Cinderella' invites without ever quite confirming the adult's interpretation of the story. But the facts of the story are clear; if it hadn't been for her fairy godmother Cinderella would never have been able to get her life started. Cinderella was, of course, ahead of her time in giving her name to a fairy tale about the contemporary 'issue' of 'reconstituted families'. Cinderella is now our contemporary and her 'issues' are our 'issues'. After all, everyone, as a child, is sometimes servile and abject and has to do what they can to get away. Just like growing up, the pursuit of pleasure is an obstacle course, and part of Cinderella's appeal is that she is a pleasure-seeker masquerading as a very helpful and cooperative person.

But as a fairy tale 'Cinderella' is also ahead of its time in that it shows us that people who have what are now euphemistically called difficult childhoods can have perfectly happy lives, can indeed live happily ever after even if they have not been happy before. All they have to do is not betray their deepest wishes. Things were certainly not looking good for Cinderella but she turned out to be extremely adept, given a little bit of help, at getting what (and where) she wanted. Indeed, the other striking thing about Cinderella – and which makes Freud's question relevant – is that men are not Cinderella's problem: women are. It is intimated in the original story that her father may have betrayed her by not protecting her from her stepmother but, ultimately, it is not finding her prince that is the problem for Cinderella, but getting to him; it's not a question of whether or not she and her prince will desire each other, but of whether she will be allowed by the other women to get to him. Both her prince and her father are captivated by the women they want, as she can't help but notice. The real problem, in other words, is not between men and women, but between women.

If only women will let them, women can get on with men. There is a scene in one of the Spencer Tracy and Katharine Hepburn films when Tracy leaves the room and Hepburn says straight to camera, 'I think men are wonderful.' No one could do this straight now, but Cinderella unequivocally thinks her prince is wonderful, and it is the other women in the story, apart from her fairy godmother, who don't want her to have that experience. As a contemporary fairy tale – which means, in the absence of alternatives, a psychological one – it is a story about why women don't want other women to have pleasure. And given that women, like their mothers, are women themselves, it is by the same token a story about how women – or parts of themselves – can be the enemies of their own desire; a story about how women, out of fear of other women's envy, want to frustrate themselves. If Cinderella's stepmother and stepsisters represent parts of herself, then they are saboteurs of her pleasure, recruited to stop her getting to the ball. The story couldn't be clearer: the ball, literally and metaphorically, is not the problem – she isn't shy or awkward, the couple clearly want each other even though they go about it in different ways, no one comes between them. Narrative is always about frustration. The story of Cinderella's life is about how she gets to have a life, about how she deals with everything and everyone that frustrates her. After that, after she marries her prince, there is no story, no need for one; they live happily ever after, which means that they get to have a life.

Even though the characters in 'Cinderella', as in all fairy stories, are not what we think of as rounded enough to be real people, the men in the story are noticeably blank. This is partly, of course, because men are the absent sex, but also because the men in the story are functional. And the function of the two main men, the father and the prince, is to be captivated (or dominated, depending on one's point of view) by their women. Cinderella's father, we assume, is so committed to his wife that he allows her to bully his daughter; and the prince clearly is not a man who has a problem committing. That women can captivate men, and vice versa, is not in question, at least in this story. Conflicts arise only between the women. Or, rather, Cinderella's wicked stepmother has created a situation in which conflict has been more or less suppressed. And it is this, of course, that makes the story, right from the start, self-evidently political; a hierarchy, a division of labour, has been established in Cinderella's home in which who is working for whom is taken for granted and so oppression is the name of the game. (It is only when Cinderella allows herself to articulate her conflict – that she wants to go to the ball and that she can't go to the ball – that the fairy godmother appears.) We know immediately that this is going to be a story about the fear of being dominated by a woman; and of what the wish to be dominated by a woman might involve. Insofar as she has let herself be bullied by her stepmother she has been free from wanting much for herself. For Cinderella, living in this regime means that she never goes out, she only works and sleeps, and no one recognizes how beautiful she is. It is, as we will see, very important in this story that the fairy godmother doesn't make Cinderella beautiful; her magic simply discloses how beautiful she is. The fabulous clothes she wears to the ball neither conceal her nor disguise her: they show her as she really is. And if adornment reveals rather than hides a woman, clarifies who she really is, then the implication is that Cinderella's abject and poorly dressed home life – if it *was* something she had imposed upon herself – was a kind of refuge; as though women can recruit other women to help them hide themselves away. As though women will do anything to avoid other women's envy. If we read the story as an internal drama – in which everyone in Cinderella's story is a part of herself – it is as though what Cinderella does, all that endless housework, is an attempt to keep at bay those female parts of herself that hate her pleasure and her pleasure-seeking because it incites envy. And it is not her pleasure that they sabotage – when she gets to her prince they have a very nice time – but her *wanting* pleasure. Her stepmother and stepsisters stop her remembering, as it were, that there are things she wants and that she is capable of having them. They come between her and her wishes, unlike her fairy godmother. Once the fairy godmother turns up, everything changes. Cinderella goes from serving her stepfamily, in an essentially self-sacrificing way, to being served, but in a notably unself-sacrificing way. It is a completely different picture of what it is to look after someone.

Cinderella's fairy godmother, rather like a certain kind of artist, enjoys nothing more than doing her work; like Picasso she doesn't seek, she finds – as if to say: what you need is always to hand if you know how to use it. The fairy godmother gets enormous pleasure from transforming the pumpkin, the rat and the mice into the coach, coachman and horses to take her to the ball. In other words, if 'Cinderella' was a story about what women want – and the evidence in the story is that it is about what Cinderella wants – the answer would be: women primarily want a mother who does everything she can (that is, magic) to facilitate their pleasure, a mother who relishes her daughter's pleasure rather than envies it or competes with it, or trivializes it. In order to pursue her pleasure a woman has to imagine that there is another woman – called a fairy godmother – who enjoys and sponsors this pleasure. In this sense her fairy godmother, in her unlikeness to her wicked stepmother, is the most important person in a girl's life. Without her, at least in the terms of the fairy tale, she can never leave home and become a woman; without this fairy godmother – the part of herself that will do whatever is necessary for her heart's desire – she will go on believing that her pleasure always harms another woman. Indeed, she could even believe that her pleasure is in harming another woman, whereas in fact this is just sometimes the consequences of following her heart's desire. So guilty is Cinderella about her own pleasure that when she does finally marry her prince she finds two 'noblemen' for her ugly stepsisters to marry.

Once Cinderella is given a bit of help by her fairy godmother she quickly gets the knack of following her heart by leaving her slipper – as good as a phone number in the circumstances – so her prince can find her. The slippers, of course, represent the couple who have to be together, but Cinderella also has a double life, or, rather, two lives which just like a pair of shoes are similar (they are both hers), and inextricable (one shoe is no good to anyone). In one life she is called Cinderella because 'when her work was finished the poor girl would sit in the chimney corner among the ashes and embers for warmth'; and in another life, which she is trying to, as it were, join up with, she is a princess 'a hundred times more beautiful than her stepsisters, although they were always magnificently dressed'. She is like an undiscovered secret; and once she is discovered the first thing she seems to learn is how to keep secrets, primarily the secret of having been to the ball. In this before-and-after story, before she was effectively lying to herself (about her beauty and her wishes), after the magic transformation she can lie to other people to protect her pleasure. She convinces her stepsisters that she hasn't been to the ball, and when they mention that the 'most beautiful princess in the world' had been there and had even sat by them 'and was very attentive', Cinderella 'feigned indifference but asked the name of the princess'. She too must be wondering what this version of herself is called, but no one knows, at least not yet. Her stepsisters, of course, tell her in detail about the ball she has supposedly missed, making oneself enviable being the last refuge of the envious. But Cinderella is now immune; coming out, being seen as she is, not trying to stop people envying her, turns out to be the best self-cure for fear of envy. The moral of the story is: girls must learn not to be intimidated by envy, not to make themselves unenviable by diminishing themselves. And this requires a certain magic, that is, a ruthless unwillingness to accept things as they are. The cure for the fear of envy is to allow oneself to be enviable. Rebels, Sartre wrote, are people who keep the world the same so they can go on rebelling against it; revolutionaries change the world. The way things were going for her, Cinderella could easily have ended up as a rebel, as a girl who can't stop complaining.

We take it for granted that the basic structure of a story is that somebody wants something and something prevents them from getting it, that in any love story there are obstacles to desire. If Cinderella so starkly asks the fundamental question – the question that makes it so contemporary – how does a girl get what she wants? – it answers the question in a very straightforward way. The problem, and the solution, is: other women. Cinderella is about the extraordinary effect that women have on other people; Cinderella's father is 'quite under the thumb' of his new wife; when Cinderella goes to the ball 'even the old king gazed on her with delight', and his son, the prince, is immediately enchanted by her. But the effect that the women have on each other is the real story of the story. And this, obviously, is one of the reasons the story works for girls. Men and women know the effect of women – what they feel in their presence – initially from their experience of their mothers. But whereas men mostly only feel the effect of women, women also grow up to have this effect. The story tells us, in its fairy-tale way, that there are two mothers, or two sides to the mother: the good mother, who to some extent sees her daughter as she is, and helps her to reveal this; and the bad mother, who treats the daughter as a usurper and rival. The bad mother says: 'You must never have what you want, and someone else must have it instead'; the good mother, the fairy godmother, says: 'My magic lets you see yourself as desirable and as desirous as you are, and you must live the life you love accordingly.' The woman who sides with the bad stepmother enjoys frustrating herself; the woman who can believe in her fairy godmother can follow her desire. For the author, and possibly the reader, of 'Cinderella' the question is not, what does a woman want? but *how* does she want? How does she go about disregarding her own wishes? What is her wanting like if she can live two such disparate lives, as drudge and princess? Drudgery, the story persuades us (and we do actually need persuading), is a bad solution to the problem of wanting. It is not satisfaction the woman fears, but the envy of her satisfaction. Men are the least of a girl's problems, at least from Cinderella's point of view.

Forsaken Favourites

What do we see in the perfect thing?

Charles Tomlinson, 'Images of Perfection'

We sometimes fall in love with people for the very things about them that will eventually drive us mad, or at least drive us away. It can seem, in retrospect, that quite unwittingly we had been doing a kind of psychic alchemy; there were things about this particular person that we were so freaked out by, that so disturbed us, we turned them into enchantments. The once charming became utterly irritating. We had come across someone – or something: a novel, a poem, a piece of music – so appalling to us that we had to get over ourselves and we called it, at the time, falling in love. Later, in the aftermath, as it were, we might think of this kind of falling in love as, say, counter-phobic, strangely self-destructive, and, so, strangely self-revealing. These are the times when falling out of love seems more interesting than falling in love, because we are not simply bereft, we are baffled; we seem to have lost something we never really wanted; we seem to have been misled.

There is, of course, always the pressure to avoid the lurking disillusionments, the bad faith of having to keep faith with oneself, of wanting to believe that all our relationships have some valuable necessity about them. These self-betrayals, if that's what they are – the loves we really regret – are tempered when we fall out of love with writers, or, rather, with their work. *What were we like if we liked this?* is a less daunting, more easily interesting question about writing that has absorbed us in the past than about lovers or friends whom we have fallen out of love with, or just lost interest in. And yet clearly our aesthetic passions are somehow of a piece with, not substitutes for or alternatives to, lovers and friends and family. The patent difference, though, is that in relationships with other people everyone is changing all the time; with writing, we change, but the words on the page don't. In this sense art never betrays us; we can only betray ourselves. *Sons and Lovers* is exactly the same book we read when we were sixteen, but we are not exactly the same person when we reread it.

Nothing reveals our resistance to giving up on past pleasures, our unwillingness to notice that we are not getting the pleasure we wanted, more than rereading the writers we loved in adolescence. These are the writers that are like lost loves, the writers who made us feel so promising, the writers who conspired with us to love our own excesses. And by the same token they are the most perilous writers to return to. 'You're the one I've been looking for/ you're the one who's got the key/ but I can't figure out whether I'm too good for you/ or you're too good for me,' Bob Dylan sings on *Street Legal*. When a writer just doesn't work for you any more, Dylan's questions are among the questions you're left with.

So when I was invited to contribute to this symposium, I was dismayed that the writer who came to mind was Dylan Thomas. A writer, it seems, I have become too good for. The poem that came immediately to mind, perhaps appropriately in the circumstances, was 'Do not go gentle into that good night', a poem that, if you grew up in Wales in the 1960s, was everywhere. I remember the revelation of reading it – or, rather, hearing it as I read it – as a fourteen-year-old; the fact that it was a poem about death wasn't a problem for me then, because I thought it was a poem about going out in the dark, something I particularly liked. I couldn't wait to go out at night, and Thomas was giving me his strange bardic encouragement. When I learned later at school what the poem was supposedly *really* about, it seemed even better: better as in deeper, graver, more portentous, more grand. And Thomas's poetry was inextricable from the legends and stories about him. Welshness was so alien to us as second-generation émigré Eastern European Jews, and Thomas made it seem all rather alluring in his slapdash, slapstick and apparently naively sophisticated Celtic fluency. If you thought, as I did then, that the Visionary Company was the only company worth keeping, Thomas was the bard of choice. Partly because he wasn't T. S. Eliot, and partly because he seemed to be the apotheosis of 'having a voice'. And also because he clearly had no idea what his poetry was about: his was an obscurity immune from academic interpretation. His seriousness, I thought then, was even greater than Arnold's, his on-the-side-of-lifeness even profounder than Lawrence's. Reading the poetry, or hearing him read it in his plummy upper-class English accent, was powerfully and obscurely moving, and left you nothing to think about.

Virtually everything that I valued as an adolescent – other than his face in Augustus John's great portrait – annoys or bores me now. His poetry seems, more often than not, like a calculated self-parody, with the joke being on us when we are moved by it. It would be more realistic to say that I let myself be tricked by Thomas's poetry; not that he, in any sense, wanted to do this to me – how could I know? – but that a sense of being tricked is what I have been left with. It is as though, in retrospect, I would like to have been more foolproof, a terrible thing to want. Clearly, we can never trust ourselves, we can only risk ourselves. Our disillusionments must be the key to our tastes. The mystery is why such vehement unmaskings are required. Why we can't just move on. Hopefully, what we learn from our mistakes is that we shall go on making them.

Acknowledgements

'Five Short Talks on Excess' were first broadcast in the BBC Radio 3 series *The Essay* and subsequently published, in a shorter version, in the *Guardian*. 'On What is Fundamental' was given as a lecture at the Columbia Psychoanalytic Society, at a conference on Fundamentalism in Brighton, and at the University of York, and published in *Salmagundi*. 'Sleeping It Off' and 'Forsaken Favourites' were published in *Three-penny Review*. 'Should School Make You Happy?' was given as a talk at King Alfred's School in London and published in a slightly different version in *Prospect*. 'The Authenticity Issue' and 'Celebrating Sebald' – first given at a conference on Sebald at the University of East Anglia – were published in *Raritan*. 'Truancy Now', 'Arbus's Freaks' (first given as a lecture at the Victoria and Albert Museum) and 'Mendelsohn's Histories' were published in the *London Review of Books*. 'On Getting Away with It' was first given as a talk at the Division 39 meeting of the APA in New York and published in *Psychoanalytic Dialogues*. 'Auden's Magic' was first given at a conference on Auden at the University of York and published in a different version in *The Reader*. Both 'Mothers and Fairy Tales' pieces were published in the *Guardian*. 'The Helpless' was given as the Townshend Lecture at Berkeley and at the University of York. 'The Lost' was given as a lecture at the San Francisco Psychoanalytic Society, the Architectural Association in London, the universities of York and of Princeton, and published in *AA Files*; otherwise 'Negative Capabilities' is previously unpublished.

I have revised each of these pieces for publication. I am very grateful to the editors of these journals, and for the invitations I have received to talk. My teaching at the University of York, where I have had wonderful colleagues and students, has been a great spur. But Judith Clark has made all the difference.